Strength Training for All Body Types

The Science of Lifting and Levers

Lee Boyce
Melody Schoenfeld

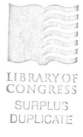

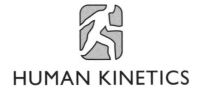

HUMAN KINETICS

Library of Congress Cataloging-in-Publication Data

Library of Congress Cataloging-in-Publication Data
Names: Boyce, Lee, 1986- author. | Schoenfeld, Melody, 1973- author.
Title: Strength training for all body types : the science of lifting and
  levers / Lee Boyce, Melody Schoenfeld.
Description: Champaign, IL : Human Kinetics, [2023] | Includes
  bibliographical references.
Identifiers: LCCN 2022018024 (print) | LCCN 2022018025 (ebook) | ISBN
  9781718212671 (paperback) | ISBN 9781718212688 (epub) | ISBN
  9781718212695 (pdf)
Subjects: LCSH: Exercise--Physiological aspects. | Human mechanics. |
  Anthropometry. | BISAC: SPORTS & RECREATION / Bodybuilding &
  Weightlifting | HEALTH & FITNESS / Exercise / General
Classification: LCC QP301 .B69 2023 (print) | LCC QP301 (ebook) | DDC
  612.7/6--dc23/eng/20220713
LC record available at https://lccn.loc.gov/2022018024
LC ebook record available at https://lccn.loc.gov/2022018025

ISBN: 978-1-7182-1267-1 (print)

Senior Acquisitions Editor: Michelle Earle; **Developmental Editor:** Anne Hall; **Managing Editor:** Kevin Matz; **Copyeditor:** Patricia L. MacDonald; **Permissions Manager:** Martha Gullo; **Graphic Designers:** Joe Buck, Julie L. Denzer; **Cover Designer:** Keri Evans; **Cover Design Specialist:** Susan Rothermel Allen; **Photograph (cover):** © Human Kinetics; **Photographs (interior):** © Human Kinetics, unless otherwise noted; **Photo Asset Manager:** Laura Fitch; **Photo Production Specialist:** Amy M. Rose; **Photo Production Manager:** Jason Allen; **Senior Art Manager:** Kelly Hendren; **Illustrations:** © Human Kinetics; **Printer:** Versa Press

Figures 5.4, 5.6, 6.9, 6.14, 7.8, 7.11, 9.11, 10.1, 10.2, 10.3, 10.8, 11.11, 12.20, 12.21, 12.30, 12.37, 12.38, 12.39 © Lee Boyce; figures 7.5, 11.13, 11.14 12.12, 12.19, 12.25 © Melody Schoenfeld.

We thank Flawless Fitness in Pasadena, CA, for assistance in providing the location for the photo shoot for this book.

Human Kinetics books are available at special discounts for bulk purchase. Special editions or book excerpts can also be created to specification. For details, contact the Special Sales Manager at Human Kinetics.

Printed in the United States of America   10 9 8 7 6 5 4 3 2 1

The paper in this book is certified under a sustainable forestry program.

Human Kinetics
1607 N. Market Street
Champaign, IL 61820
USA

United States and International
Website: **US.HumanKinetics.com**
Email: info@hkusa.com
Phone: 1-800-747-4457

Canada
Website: **Canada.HumanKinetics.com**
Email: info@hkcanada.com

E8594

Tell us what you think!
Human Kinetics would love to hear what we can do to improve the customer experience. Use this QR code to take our brief survey.

Contents

Exercise Finder

DEADLIFT EXERCISES

Exercise name	Body type	Page #
Conventional deadlift	Long torso, long arms, large hands	67
Trap bar deadlifts	Short torso, long legs; tall	71
Deadlift from blocks	Short torso, long legs; tall; limited mobility	72
Paused deadlift	Short torso, long legs; tall	72
Isometric deadlift	Short torso, long legs; tall	73
Eccentric-free deadlifts (touch-and-go and dead-stop methods)	Short torso, long legs; tall	74
Medium sumo barbell deadlift	Big all over	77
Kettlebell deadlift	Big all over	79
Deficit deadlift	Short	80
Snatch grip deadlift	Short	82
Hip rockbacks	All	85
Dowel hinge pattern	All	85
Glute bridge	All	85

SQUAT EXERCISES

Exercise name	Body type	Page #
Barbell back squat	Long torso, short legs	87
Barbell front squat	Short torso, long legs; long femurs; tall	89
Foam roller extensions	Limited upper body mobility	90
Front squat with lifting straps	Big all over; limited mobility	91
Heels-elevated dumbbell squat	Tall; long legs, long femurs	91
Slow, eccentric paused back squat	Long shins; short	93
Isometric squat	Long shins; short	94
Safety bar squat	Big all over; limited mobility	95
Frankenstein squat	Big all over; limited mobility	97
Hip belt squat	Big all over; limited mobility	98
Weight belt squat	Big all over; limited mobility	99
Box squat with lower bar position	Tall; long legs, long femurs	100
Free barbell squat to parallel depth	Tall; long legs, long femurs	101
Chain or banded squat	Lifters with bad knees	102
Band target squat	Lifters with bad knees	103

BENCH PRESS EXERCISES

Exercise name	Body type	Page #
Standard bench press	Short arms; big all over	107
Bench press with tucked feet	Long arms; slender torso	109

BENCH PRESS EXERCISES *(continued)*

Exercise name	Body type	Page #
Wide-grip bench press	Long arms; slender torso; anyone needing strength in the upper portion of the press	109
Floor press	Long arms; slender torso; anyone needing strength in the upper portion of the press	110
Pin press	Long arms; slender torso; anyone needing strength in the upper portion of the press	110
Chains or banded bench press	Long arms; slender torso; anyone needing strength in the upper portion of the press	111
Board press	Long arms; slender torso; anyone needing strength in the upper portion of the press	112
Reverse banded bench press	Long arms; slender torso; anyone needing strength in the upper portion of the press	113
1.5 repetition bench press	Long arms; slender torso	114
Close-grip bench press	Long arms; slender torso	115
Incline bench press	All	116
Supinated-grip bench press	Shoulder injuries; weak wrists	118
Paused bench press	Short arms; big all over	120
Dumbbell or kettlebell bench press	Short arms; big all over	119
Cambered bar press	Short arms; big all over	120
Multigrip barbell bench press	All	122

OVERHEAD PRESS EXERCISES

Exercise name	Body type	Page #
Standard overhead press	Short arms or long arms and high muscle mass; short torso	123
Strict press	Long arms	124
Landmine press	Long arms	125
Seated press	Long torso	126
Z press	Long torso	127
Dumbbell press	Long arms	128
Pin press	Long arms	128
Push press	Long arms	129
Trap bar pin press	Big all over	129
Log press	Big all over	130
Pressing against pins	Short arms	131

(continued)

CHIN-UP EXERCISES

Exercise name	Body type	Page #
Standard chin-up	Short	134
Flexed arm hang	Tall; long arms	137
Rack chin-up	Tall; long arms	138
Eccentric chin-up	Big all over	139
Neutral-grip chin-up	Big all over	142
Ring chin-up	Big all over	142
Band-assisted chin-up	Big all over	144
Sternum chin-up or pull-up	Short; short arms	146
Band-assisted single-arm chin-up	Short; short arms	147
Weighted chin-up	Short; short arms	148
Band-resisted chin-up	Short; short arms	149

ROW EXERCISES

Exercise name	Body type	Page #
Seated cable row with V-grip	Narrow shoulders	151
Wide-grip seated row	Wide shoulders; wide torso	154
Barbell bent-over row	Long torso, short arms, short legs	155
Single-arm dumbbell row	Long torso, short legs	156
Row with adjustable bench	Long torso, short legs	159
Ring inverted row	Big all over	160
Heels-elevated ring row	Big all over	162
Pendlay row	Long legs, short torso	164
Modified Pendlay row	Long legs; limited mobility	165
T-bar row	Long legs; limited mobility	165
Band-resisted row	Small hands	167

ABDOMINAL EXERCISES

Exercise name	Body type	Page #
Thoracic rotation	Big all over; limited mobility	170
Supine spinal rotation	Big all over	171
Foam roller thoracic extensions	All	172
Wheel rollouts	Big all over	172
Suspension trainer standing rollout	Big all over; long arms	173
Inchworms	Big all over; long limbs	173
Long-arm sit-up	Long arms	175
Pallof press	Long arms	176
Alternate leg lowering	Long legs	177
Hanging knee raise	Long legs	178
Weighted carries	Small hands	179

ABDOMINAL EXERCISES *(continued)*

Exercise name	Body type	Page #
Captain's chair exercise	Small hands	180
Decline leg raise	Small hands, short arms	181
Mountain climber	All	182
Supine Chinese plank	All	183
Prone Chinese plank	All	183

ACCESSORY WORK

Exercise name	Body type	Page #
Tate press	All	188
Overhead triceps extension	All	189
Triceps press-down	All	190
JM press	All	191
Plyometric push-up	All	192
Push-up with dumbbells	All	193
Narrow-stance push-up	All	194
Wide-stance push-up	All	194
Bench dip	All	194
Vertical dip	All	195
Dumbbell and machine flys	All	197
Cable crossover	All	198
Cuban press	All	198
Dumbbell lateral raise	All	199
Standard barbell curl	All	201
Standard dumbbell curl	All	201
Standard EZ-bar curl	All	201
Hammer curl	All	201
Reverse curl	All	202
Zottman curl	All	202
Reverse-grip bent-over row	All	202
Yates row	Long shins; long femurs	205
Kettlebell row	Long legs	205
Drag curl	All	206
Dumbbell snatch	All	206
Lat pull-down	All	208
Leg press	All	209
Walking lunge	All	211
Staggered-stance single-leg deadlift	All	215
Bent-leg single-leg deadlift	All	215

(continued)

ACCESSORY WORK *(continued)*

Exercise name	Body type	Page #
Straight-leg single-leg deadlift	All	215
Eccentric Nordic curl	All	216
Nordic curl hip hinge	All	217
Reverse Nordic curl	All	219
Reverse hyperextensions	All	221
Rear-foot-elevated split squat	All	222
Rear-foot-elevated split squat with deficit	Short	224
Straight-legged Copenhagen plank	Short; long torso, short legs	226
Bent-legged Copenhagen plank	Big all over; long legs	227
Cossack squat	All	228
Box Cossack squat	Big all over; tall	229
Barbell hip thrust	All	230
Cable pull-through	All	230
Leg extensions	All	231
Leg curls	All	232

Foreword

"Nothing good comes easy. If it did, everyone would have it."

It's a memory I won't shake. My first time in an NBA weight room, I was nothing short of impressed. I was newly signed by the Lakers, and in that training center, all the guys were there to work. Nothing more and nothing less. I made sure I held my own. We would come in, do our exercises, and not bat an eye about the difficulty or volume our coach asked of us. Everyone had his own program, because everyone is different. Not only were there different demands due to our positions on the court, but we also had different levels of fitness, different bodies, different needs, and different injuries to bear in mind.

I was excited for my first pro season. And I have remembered that quote until this day.

Even more important, I was impressed to see the machines built for someone like me—taller athletes with longer limbs. And that was really cool. The equipment was nothing you'd find at your average Gold's Gym up the street. This couldn't have been better for me as a 7 footer with a 7'1" wingspan. I had no problem building muscle; I've always been a bigger guy, so that part of my training wasn't hard. My struggle came from having access to the right equipment and the right programming at all times. (Props to my strength coaches for all the help there.) There were other guys in the weight room who didn't feel they needed to be in there. They were ready to work, but in truth they could not stand lifting—especially compared to playing ball or doing drills—so they saw less of a point. Everyone is different, and we all need individualized programs to maintain proper conditioning.

I think because I loved lifting, it was easy for me to be in the weight room. I enjoyed being in there, and it was fun to go after the heavy stuff and chase size and strength gains. But I noticed later in my career that things began to change. I had different needs in order to keep performing well. I was already big, and I didn't need to get any bigger. I just needed to maintain. By this point, I needed to focus on other things like calisthenics and to prioritize my mobility and flexibility to keep my joints healthy. I couldn't hammer away at big lifts day in and day out because of how much my levers had to handle compared to the next guy. I started incorporating different methods like yoga to stay limber and loose. Like I said, everyone needs individualized training, and that adjustment to my focus is what worked for *me*.

In the league, you might have one guy who's bowlegged, another guy who's all legs and arms, and another guy who's knock-kneed. You can't expect those athletes to train the same. And I know for sure that most bigs in the league have bad feet—something that for me required more attention, stretching, and tissue work. When you have a shorter guard who's 180 pounds training with a man who's my height and weighs 265 pounds, a lot needs to be considered in the weight room to help both of their games improve.

That's why this book Lee and Melody have written is a really valuable resource in a world where very little literature exists on the subject of weight training and body types. I can think of lots of places a guide like this could have been helpful in the training world 10 or 15 years ago, especially for ball players. But whether you're a pro athlete or a total beginner, it's important to know just where you fall on the spectrum. Just because you don't play a sport, it doesn't mean those needs disappear. Everyone can take something positive away from what the authors have put together here, so enjoy this read. You'll be coming back to it over and over.

—Robert Sacre, Los Angeles Lakers Center (2012-2016)

Acknowledgments

Having spoken and written about this subject matter for years, and being a walking, talking example of a whole lot of what's contained in these pages, I think it's safe to say this is a topic that's close to home for me. Melody Schoenfeld is an efficient, research-driven strength coach/workhorse/mastermind whom I had instant chemistry with from the moment we met. And she too is a walking, talking example of what's contained in these pages. The two of us joining forces was the perfect combination. I can't think of any other partner and coauthor this would have worked with. I'm still surprised and impressed that she could handle my fastidiousness. She deserves maximum thanks for her brilliance—and for being just plain awesome.

I've made a lot of great friends in the fitness industry over the last 15 years, a number of whom have been pivotal in making this project possible. Huge thanks are in order for Tim DiFrancesco, Joe DeFranco, Scott Douglas (and all the folks over at the NSCA), Jay King, Ricky Jacques, Eric Wong Kai Pun, Natalie Saccucci, Eb Samuel, Adam Firer, Eric Smith, Kris Raghubir, Lee Janota, Andrew Coates, and Gursharon Kaur for their support, time, and help in various ways throughout this process. Human Kinetics knows how to get the job done, and I can't thank them enough for liking this idea enough to give it the green light and get behind it for publishing. To everyone involved—the editors, photographers, and any other staff who may have been involved with making this happen—thank you. A special shout out to Rob Sacre for gifting us with a gem of a foreword for this book, which truly put the icing on the cake. Our book was a long time coming, and it was a long process that was never ever boring or stale. It still feels like just the other day when I walked into my first commercial gym workplace as a new hire to train my first client, back in 2007. That same day, I decided there was no turning back. Mom, this one's for you.

—Lee Boyce

This book was a love letter to the diversity in bodies that sorely needed to be written, and I could not have asked for a better partner in crime to do this with than the very awesome, very tall, and very smart Lee Boyce. I also want to thank Lou Schuler and Nick Bromberg for hosting The Fitness Summit for so many years—Lee and I crossed paths because of it, and I met so many other amazing people as a result of speaking at and attending that conference. Tremendous thanks to Michelle Earle, Roger Earle, Anne Hall, and the rest of the staff at Human Kinetics for putting their faith in this book and putting up with our endless revisions. A big thank you to Lee Janota for all the support throughout the writing of this book. And an extra-special thank you to my brother, Brad, for always encouraging me; without him, I never would have even thought about entering the fitness world in the first place.

—Melody Schoenfeld

A huge thank you to our friends, colleagues, and clients who volunteered their time, energy, and good looks to the photographs in this book: Odd Haugen, Lee Janota, Aaron Anderson, Sally Lewis, Wenona Cole-McLaughlin, Bill Hada, Erin Kurasz, Ken Kurasz, Bryan Sanchez, Sicily Easley, Kimzey McGrath, Michael Witt, Will Guiliani, Brenda Garcia Davidge, Eric Smith, and Roberta Tragarz.

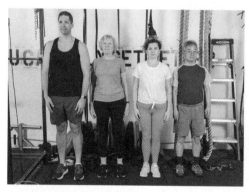

Left to right: Aaron Anderson, fitness enthusiast; Sally Lewis, dog agility handler; Wenona Cole-McLaughlin, fitness enthusiast; Bill Hada, fitness enthusiast.

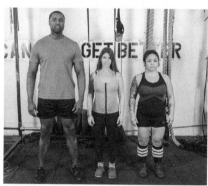

Left to right: Lee Boyce, track sprinter and jumper; Melody Schoenfeld, strongman, grip athlete, and mas wrestler; Sicily Easley, powerlifter.

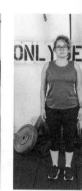

Brenda Garci Davidge, roller derby at

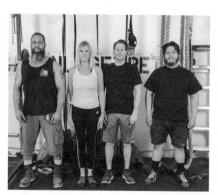

Left to right: Lee Janota, strongman, grip athlete, and Highland Games athlete; Erin Kurasz, law enforcement officer; Ken Kurasz, fitness enthusiast; Bryan Sanchez, strongman.

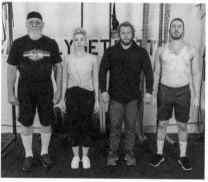

Left to right: Odd Haugen, strongman, grip athlete, and mas wrestler; Kimzey McGrath, fitness enthusiast; Michael Witt, strongman, grip athlete, and mas wrestler; Will Guiliani, grip athlete.

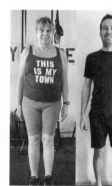

Roberta Tragarz and Smith, fitness ethus

Introduction

"My body doesn't do that."

If you've ever worked with clients, or even just listened to conversations at the gym, you've more than likely heard someone say something like that. Many of the cues trainers have been taught in whatever education we've had simply don't work on all people. And there's a reason for that:

Human bodies don't all present the same way.

I know. Shocking. But still, it stands to reason that telling someone to get their shins parallel to the ground in a deadlift isn't going to happen for some people.

The geometry of the human body plays a huge role in how a person might excel—or, conversely, perform really poorly—at any given movement. Our different joint angles, bone lengths, and overall structures may mean that certain lifts might be much more of a challenge, but it doesn't necessarily mean that those lifts cannot or should not be performed. It may just take a little form tweaking in order to make them the best they can be.

This book explores and celebrates the differences in moving bodies. In it, we break down the ways unique bodies manage various lifts, and we discuss how to best take advantage of a given set of levers (i.e., arms, legs, torso) in order to optimize those lifts. Using a mixture of physics, biomechanics, geometry, and personal experience, we hope to create a comprehensive guide to training bodies of all kinds in the ways they move best.

The reality of the situation is this: When you take a closer look at every sport, especially at the elite levels of competition, you'll without a doubt begin to see a trend. Body types become a bit more homogenous because certain bodies are going to better cater to the requirements and demands of that sport. Strangely, no one's ever taken the same closer look at lifting for performance. The fact of the matter is, not everyone is perfectly built for lifting. But everyone still needs to lift.

That certain body types are more suited to elite lifting may hold true in a standardized competition, but when it comes to training in the general sense, we all have the chance to level the playing field by making adjustments to suit our needs.

Strength training is something everyone should do, but it's not something everyone's built for if we're stuck within the confines of conventional movement patterns and fixed programs and techniques. It's not a one size fits all. Moreover, in sports, an athlete has no choice but to adapt to what's being asked of them. Like jumping high enough to dunk a basketball no matter whether you're tall or short. Or hitting a home run whether you've got a long reach or a short one. We don't have the power to make modifications in that world, and it becomes survival of the fittest in terms of body type to separate the elite from the mediocre. Training doesn't need to be that way.

It's about recognizing *new* standards for strength and program design that can keep various body types safe while making them strong—even if that means rewriting a few rules you read in your training textbook along the way.

Let's face it. Lifting is not a one-size-fits-all endeavor. Let's not treat it as such.

PART I

Foundations

The first four chapters of this book will set the tone for the content we're discussing and remind you that a trainer should consider the uniqueness of the individual as it pertains to training. It is important to think in many shades of grey rather than in black and white. "It depends" is a very real and valid answer for many questions regarding technique, exercise prescription, and program design.

In the real world, there is variety in human body types, and an individual's body type can largely influence their ceiling of potential in a given endeavor. In many cases, it can even influence which endeavors a person will opt to practice the most. Learning about basic physical principles like shear, work, or torque in a clear and comprehensive way can make the concepts understandable so they can be accurately applied in later chapters.

How are we *supposed* to train? Isolation training like a physique competitor? Compound movements like a sports athlete? What about locomotive strongman-style work? If there's anything that tends to cause the most contention in the world of fitness and strength training, it's this topic. Everywhere you turn, you'll find a different answer to the question of how to train. The arguments run rampant, and we're here to give you a spoiler: We aren't about to participate in these debates.

What we *will* do is establish common ground with fundamental movement patterns. This way, regardless of what method of training an individual is involved in, it will be able to be categorized and analyzed. Looking at *patterns*, rather than muscles, opens the door for many variations of a given exercise to fit. It's also a good starting point to build a discussion around.

As you explore the first four chapters of this book, allow them to open your mind—they will likely lead you to question the rules you've accepted as hard, fast, and unbreakable. We start with setting the foundation for what's to come by using a little history, a little science, a little theory, and a sprinkling of our favorite ingredient—common sense.

Chapter 1

The Importance of Body Type Specificity

The human body's ideal proportions have long been a topic of discussion from the standpoint of aesthetics. Symmetry has often been seen as an ideal, as demonstrated by Leonardo da Vinci's *Vitruvian Man*, whose proportions allowed him to fit neatly into a circle.

In life, however, most humans are not so symmetrical. The median height of men in North America, Australia, Europe, and East Asia is a little over 5 feet, 10 inches, while the median height for women is a little under 5 foot 5 (Roser 2013). A large percentage of individuals fall above and below that median line, and within all of that, there are varying degrees of limb lengths, torso lengths, shoulder widths, waist-to-hip ratios, and so forth.

There isn't currently a standard measure of body proportions. However, some measures, such as leg length, are used to determine illness and growth patterns. Leg length is of particular importance for movement—legs should be around 50 percent of total height in order to be most efficient at traveling on two legs (Bogin 2010). Human proportions are also useful for such things as regulating temperature, carrying things with the arms and hands, gesturing and other forms of nonverbal communication, and running long distances (Bogin 2010).

Human proportions, height, and mass are affected by a number of factors, not least among them environment. In colder climates, having shorter limbs and larger body mass can help preserve warmth, while in warmer regions, long limbs and bodies can help prevent overheating (Ruff 2002). Nutrition also plays a strong role in development, with malnutrition causing issues with growth and limb length, and overnutrition adding to total girth (Azcorra, 2013)).

In short, there is no ideal human proportion, considering all the factors involved with the human body's makeup. There are, however, certain body proportions that prove advantageous to particular movements, and others that can pose more of a problem. It therefore becomes necessary to manipulate biomechanics in order to optimize performance for various body types in different areas of strength, conditioning, and sport.

Problems may arise for, for instance, taller athletes who deadlift—because the bar must travel for a longer trajectory, and more strain is placed on the lower back for a longer time than for a shorter athlete.

Conversely, a short, light athlete might be at a great disadvantage for many strongman events. The power stair, for instance, requires the ability to deadlift a weight past the normal height, and a shorter athlete might need to perform some pretty impressive feats of extension in order to get the weight stack onto the step. Additionally, a light weight can make it more difficult to put on more muscle and in general provides a lower overall strength capacity—there are simply some weights a light athlete is unlikely to be able to lift.

Having short arms can impede throwing distance and velocity in throwing sports, so shorter-armed athletes will need to find alternative techniques in order to optimize throwing power. Meanwhile, long legs can create much slower turnover, reaction time, and acceleration when sprinting, so a long-legged sprinter might have to train quite differently from a shorter-legged sprinter in order to improve in these areas.

To date, there are few studies pertaining specifically to the effects of body type and limb length on sport performance. Those that exist tend to be very sport specific. A handful of studies have been performed on limb length and sport performance in volleyball (Aouadi et al. 2012), swimming (Nevill et al. 2015), handball (Sarvestan et al. 2019), and some other sports. A few studies are specific to weightlifting (Musser et al. 2014; Vidal et al. 2021) and powerlifting (Justin et al. 2007; Keogh et al. 2009). A systematic review has been done of the current studies on limb asymmetries and sport performance (Bishop et al. 2018). This is clearly an area in need of more research.

There is, to our knowledge, no literature addressing this subject in educational materials for coaches and trainers or in mainstream materials. This is a void that we feel needs to be filled. Coaches will manage a tremendous variety of body types, many of which may not fit the ideal for that particular sport. The training for nonideal body types may look quite different from that for more conventionally bodied athletes. Understanding how each person can use their proportions to their best advantage will help create better athletes. And that, after all, is a coach's main focus.

Programming: The Five Overlooked Factors for Success

Knowing how to bring out the best in each body type is what will differentiate a good coach with good programming from an average or poor coach with generic, cookie-cutter methods. Perusing the Internet to find a program that may be respectable by all standards is only as good as the athlete who performs it. And programs tend to assume the best of an individual—as they should. The program (and its creator) can't see the lifter. The only thing it has to go on is the general track record of the lifts prescribed as far as the history of the general public. Here are examples of what a generic program intended for mass consumption can overlook.

A Lifter's Real Age

The calendar age of a lifter needs to be considered when embarking on a strength training program involving resistance. Consider an example: You can take great care of a 1974 Shelby GT, having given it its scheduled maintenance right on time, updated its parts, and so on, and you can likely get a lot out of that vehicle on the road because of how well it's been maintained. However, if you expect that 1974 Shelby GT to beat out a 2020 Shelby GT, you can bet that 9 times out of 10 it will be outperformed. The simple reason is that it's a vehicle that needs more attention, because it possesses an engine that has more mileage on it. The engine has turned over that many more times, and the axles have rotated for millions more revolutions. It may even need more time warming up before driving—especially depending on the driving conditions. There's no disputing this truth. It's a *used* vehicle.

Hackneyed as it is to use the old car analogy, it fits. The human body can be viewed in a similar way, and the previous example is probably brimming with linkages. You can't expect to push a 48-year-old body to the same degree (or frequency) that you push a 20-year-old body. Nor can you expect it to recover at the same rate. If this were true and possible, there would be no retirement age range in professional sports (most usually between 35 and 40 years), and athletes would be breaking records into their 50s and beyond. A training program for sale on the Internet or by way of a textbook doesn't know the age of the individual attempting its workouts. Whether the prescriptions and parameters are too intense or the wrong overall fit for the lifter is left to chance.

A Lifter's Training Age

Contrary to calendar age, the *training* age refers to how many years a lifter has spent exposed to results-oriented training methodologies. A 20-year-old varsity water polo athlete who's been working out in the weight room for enhanced performance since age 17 would have a training age of 3. A 49-year-old financial advisor who was sedentary his entire life until finally hiring a personal trainer after his 47th birthday would have a training age of only 2, despite having more than twice the calendar age of the water polo athlete.

Adversely, if that water polo player from the first example never stopped training, he'd eventually have a training age of 32 by the time he reached the age of our financial advisor. How elaborate the programming is, including its overall difficulty level and complexity of individual exercises (for instance, an Olympic clean or snatch compared with a simple row or curl), can have a serious impact on the training effect delivered by the workouts themselves; one prescription may not be as suited to a given individual based on their training age or overall weight training experience.

On the same note, a trainee's skill level usually goes hand in hand with that trainee's training age. How easily an experienced lifter will pick up a new movement pattern compared with someone with limited training experience or low body awareness can be a major factor as to how well suited a program may be for the individual, and it can have an impact on the results they receive as a by-product. On the flip side, a lifter with a great deal of skill in a movement may not receive all the same benefits of the pattern (depending on the goals of the individual) because of how efficiently the lifter may move under load when performing a set of reps. If the movement is one that's been practiced with good form for years, the trade-off between strength and fitness-related results will make itself known by way of the law of diminishing returns (simply put, the more practice you have with something—in this case, a lifting movement—the less value you'll receive from it over time). Progressive overload may present additional challenge and benefit, but there are a few caveats that may not always make added weight the desired primary area of focus. More on that later.

A Lifter's Injury History

Prescribing barbell squats to a daily max—a staple of the Bulgarian training method—would be a respectable choice for an individual looking to improve the strength and size of their legs over the duration of a periodized training program, with all things equal. However, prescribing squats to an individual who's had a bilateral patellar tendon rupture and hernia surgery, and suffers from discogenic back issues, would cause plenty of ambivalence. Any good trainer would be diligent to understand their athletes' history, including wear and tear on joints, chronic pain, acute injuries, or surgeries that sidelined training progress. The answer isn't always to remove the training protocol entirely, but it could mean adjusting the programming to better suit the needs of the individual.

In the case of the lifter with the knee ruptures, repaired hernia, and back issues, barbell squatting might not be off the table entirely, but a reduced lifting volume, a greater number of ramping sets, lower daily max thresholds, longer rest periods, a reduced weekly squatting frequency, and a better gauge on perceived exertion levels would be worthwhile in this case, and very effective anecdotally speaking—especially since the lifter in this example is one of the authors.

A Lifter's Anthropometry and Size

You may have assumed this to be the next area of focus, and it makes perfect sense. As you'll see in chapter 4, strength training as a whole has much less to do with muscles and much more to do with understanding physics. How loading acts on joints throughout the body that are meant to bear such load is contingent on the leverages the body possesses. To expect the same results of a lifter who has a 28-inch leg length compared with a lifter with a 37-inch leg length when putting them through the same lower body workout would be dismissive of the fact that individual anthropometry requires individualized attention.

As you'll see in the next chapter, the body type is what creates the natural baseline for high performance in a sport or discipline, and any outliers to this rule are usually faced with a greater hill to climb to achieve the same standard of performance. A bench press will act differently on the shoulders of a 6-foot-tall individual with a wingspan of 5 feet, 11 inches compared with that of a 6-foot-tall individual with a wingspan of 6 feet, 7 inches. Other unchangeable skeletal norms should also be taken into consideration, such as the positioning of a lifter's hip sockets (acetabula) on the pelvis (figure 1.1) and how such variety can influence the training effect of patterns like deadlifts and squats and their variations.

Whether the goal is building muscle, burning fat, increasing strength, or improving conditioning, it's important to know that one size does not fit all.

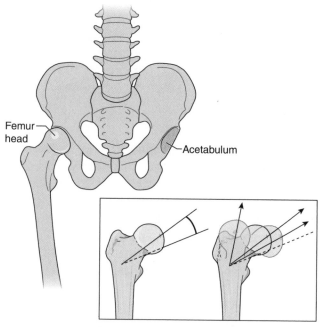

FIGURE 1.1 Hip socket configurations.

What Is Strength?

Let's begin by explaining what strength isn't—and in doing so, show where the strength and conditioning world can tend to drop the ball.

Strength is *not* fitness.

Strength, in its most simplistic form, is the ability to move heavy things by applying forces against resistances. Possessing strength is one of the most important attributes of a healthy body, if not the most important, but it is merely one component of fitness. For many, this reality is foreign territory. As a result, many trainers unwittingly coach their general population clients to become powerlifters by default—focusing too much on their max efforts and traditional barbell movements with progressive overload . . . and nothing else.

In reality, there are 11 components of fitness that cover both health and skill. Strength is one of the 11. In other words, strength indeed is not fitness—it's about 9 percent of fitness. Let's review the other 10 components of fitness to make sure we're at the same starting point. If we're going to talk about training for fitness, it's worth getting a proper, rounded, and whole assessment of what fitness is, for better or worse—regardless of personal biases toward certain aspects of it.

Speed

Speed refers to how quickly you can move your body parts in space (individually or together) from one place to another. Measuring speed, or the production of velocity, typically involves measuring the ratio of the distance an object (including the body) travels over the time it takes to get there. Typical units of measurement include meters per second, kilometers per hour, and miles per hour. Someone running the 100-meter dash in 10 seconds has an average speed of 10 meters per second.

Power

Power combines strength with speed to find the key intersection of force and velocity production. Many people mistakenly think training power involves lifting as heavy as possible—likely thanks to the title of *powerlifting* and the tenets of that sport. In truth, the implement being lifted needs to be light enough to be accelerated; using medicine balls and kettlebells, performing Olympic lifts with light weights, and doing plyometrics are all effective ways to train power. A powerful individual has well-trained fast-twitch muscle fibers and a good base of strength to make their muscles contract at a very rapid rate.

Cardiorespiratory Capacity

Mentioned earlier, the strength and conditioning world can place less than appropriate emphasis on certain capacities of human fitness, and this would certainly be one of the leading categories. Things like a person's $\dot{V}O_2$max (or the amount of oxygen a person's muscles can use when training), cardiac output, and stroke volume matter for overall health, and the most effective way to improve these measures is steady-state cardiorespiratory training.

Reaction Time

Your reflexes affect you in different areas of your life—from reacting to a starter's pistol on the diving block at a swim meet to quickly hitting the brakes when a car ahead of you swerves off course. There are limited exercises involving weights that can help develop this capacity. Reaction time may seem like a less important attribute to a resistance trainee, since most of lifting occurs in a much more controlled and less dynamic environment with fewer athletic demands. However, certain variations of lifts, such as explosive training and Olympic lifting, hinge greatly on timing for proper movement quality. The ability to know exactly when to synchronize the body with a catch position for a push press or jerk pattern (as an example) involves some reaction to the bar's travel and forces. Moreover, on the eccentric (or negative) phases of many lifts, this attribute will come in handy to control the bar to the body or floor. In the event of a mistake, slip, or poorly timed rep, having fast reaction time can help prevent injury.

Muscular Endurance

This category is often confused with cardiorespiratory capacity, since training for aerobic fitness involves exploiting your muscular endurance to remain in motion over extended periods. Training muscular endurance puts your muscles to work under a secondary energy system known as glycolysis. The muscles operate with the assistance of oxygenated blood being pumped to the muscles—unlike anaerobic training such as sprinting or plyometrics, which operates without any oxygen and has a much earlier fatigue threshold. The ability to make muscles contract repeatedly is a product of good muscular endurance, and the nature of our day-to-day lives suggests certain muscles and structures of our bodies will rely much more on muscular endurance than others.

Flexibility

The ability to lengthen muscle tissue to change a joint's position may be underrated in the world of strength training, but it doesn't mean it's a useless attribute. This capacity, along with many others, reduces with age—making flexibility training important to practice. A stronger muscle may be able to contract more forcefully, but turning that into ideal mobility will depend on how much the antagonistic (or opposing) muscle can stretch to open up the other side. To think about this in practice, lie on your back with your hands by your sides. Lift one straight leg as far as it will go. This simultaneously relies on the contraction strength of your hip flexor group and rectus femoris quadriceps muscle *and* the flexibility of your hamstrings group and gluteal muscles on the back of the same leg. When it's all put together, it gives a good indication of what the mobility of the hip joint looks like through the action of active hip flexion. Simply put, without flexibility, you can't get mobile. Training without mobility will set the stage for inevitable injuries or chronic pain in your near future.

Body Composition

Especially lately, this aspect of health-related fitness has become one of the more popularly talked about and scrutinized. But speaking objectively, it's important to avoid euphemisms and call a spade a spade. Body composition—more specifically the ratio of lean tissue to fat tissue—needs to be in an optimal range to support long-term health. Of course, this will vary from person to person depending on certain factors, but countless research indicates that obesity has linkages to diabetes, hypertension, stroke, cardiovascular disease, and more. There's a fine line between embracing a body in any shape or size while making the evergreen goal of *improved fitness* (remember, body composition is a component of fitness, so improved fitness in this case would mean improving that composition) versus using that mindset to shirk the responsibility of doing so because of an assumed disposition of mental calm. It's very important to pursue all aspects of fitness, and to prioritize those aspects to what fits the individual's greatest needs the most urgently. An impressive deadlift or squat may be commendable, but it won't save your heart from cardiac arrest due to high cholesterol levels, poor nutritional choices, and a lack of aerobic practice. As far as obesity goes, in the United States, it's not a problem that's been solved—far from it. In fact, numbers are trending upward. The worst thing to hinder addressing and solving a growing health problem is to not consider it a problem at all.

Agility

The ability to change directions in a hurry by use of fast footwork relies heavily on the contractile strength of the muscles and the health of the connective tissue—the tendons and ligaments that hold bones and muscles in articulation. Being agile means being able to decelerate rapidly, cut hard, and change body orientation in the blink of an eye. Agility combines speed with power and quickness, and training for it involves a departure from strictly weight room sagittal plane exercise selections. Becoming stronger in classic compound movements like the overhead press, squat, chin-up, and deadlift can improve bone density and strength, but it won't have much of an effect on agility, since each of these movements is performed in the sagittal plane. Getting onto a soccer or football field and exploring patterns of forward-to-backward and side-to-side running, jumping, and sprinting movements would be a better way to work on this attribute.

Balance

Interestingly, balance is often linked directly to core training, and it's a definite reason the unstable surface training trend of the mid 2000s picked up steam and BOSU balls, rocker boards, Swiss balls, and more became the most trendy gym equipment to possess. Having good balance does involve some core strength, but more than direct strength work, it relies on proprioception and spatial awareness. As a person ages and their musculoskeletal system doesn't perform the way it used to, balance becomes one of the attributes of fitness that is compromised. Being proprioceptive indicates that a person has a good handle on their limb position in space, which having good balance basically epitomizes. Think about a tightrope walker performing a feat, 20 stories off the ground. The tightrope is in their direct line of sight, and the ground is hundreds of feet below, which can really throw off one's perspective and frame of reference. Thanks to strong proprioceptive skills, the tightrope walker doesn't let these things interfere with the steady control of their arms and legs to prevent them from losing balance and falling off the rope.

Here's the thing—training for proprioception (and ultimately balance) involves training on unstable surfaces or compromised bases of support. And a simple law of the universe is this: You cannot produce maximal force against an unstable surface. If you could, athletes might record the highest vertical jumps and fastest 40-yard dash times on the beach in sand rather than on flat, solid ground. Knowing this, it's clear that balance deserves its own dedicated approach to training in the gym, and conventional methods may not do the job.

Coordination

To piggyback off of balance, coordination demands that the brain and the muscles work harmoniously. Successfully achieving this will result in the limbs working independently of one another, especially relative to the trunk. The ability of the brain to tell the hand to do something different from the foot, or of the eye to synchronize actions with the extremities, is the baseline for basic prowess in most sports. To an extent, it's a requirement for proper function and safety when lifting weights. Coordination can exist among the limbs while moving the body or when dealing with an external load (like a basketball, a soccer ball, or even a loaded barbell).

How Strong Do You Need to Be?

You may have guessed this was the question we were building up to.

Although the next chapter will dive into this subject a bit more directly, it's good to start thinking about the double-edged sword that is strength training. It is indeed beneficial for becoming stronger, but it can come at the expense of other elements of fitness if excessive amounts of time are spent strictly strength training. When making strength the focus, there may be some residual benefit to *some* of the other 10 components of fitness, but in many cases, a decrease will be noticed since those areas no longer receive a lifter's attention. Seeing results in a component of fitness requires performing a higher volume of movements that are pertinent to the goal in question. In the case of strength training, you won't get very far if the exercises you've selected as the core of your program are biceps curls, calf raises, pec deck flys, and press-downs. Strength is dictated by the central nervous system, and for that reason, compound lifts with appreciable load are the smartest ways to train for it. Force production involves joints of the body working in harmony with one another to produce effort from the entire body, which is why it's generally agreed that lifts like squats, deadlifts, overhead presses, chin-ups, and bench presses are among the wisest choices in general for trackable and sustainable improvements in strength.

With that said, when the majority of an athlete's training volume gets devoted to movements like these, it can leave little to no time for other accessory movements, let alone other attributes of fitness. It's a safe assumption that excessive strength training over an extended period will put a damper on progression of muscular endurance, cardiorespiratory capacity, and likely flexibility, to name a few. By extension, training exclusively to get stronger is typically augmented by eating in a caloric surplus. To develop more absolute strength (a term you'll be familiarized with in the next chapter), it helps to carry more surface area to move greater loads—a reason lifters with the heaviest powerlifts ever recorded are all very large men, and not built like sprinters or gymnasts. So inevitably, another area of fitness that often gets compromised from an extended focus on exclusively strength training would be body composition.

Knowing about these often-seen training trade-offs plants the seed that the information contained in these pages should be taken for what it is—and that the bigger picture and broader scope of training for proper fitness and health should not be lost. The strength and conditioning world indeed drops the ball when the *conditioning* part of *strength and conditioning* falls by the wayside in favor of a new personal record. Similarly, understanding that workouts can be tailored and modified to properly cater to varying body types doesn't mean applying them just to strength workouts. Conditioning workouts, cardiorespiratory workouts, and even body-weight training can all benefit from looking at biomechanics through a more dissecting lens.

In a similar vein, many recreational lifters have the goal of training for physique. Coaches who work with such clients often deliver programming and instruction that place more of a focus on performance than aesthetic advancements. The age-old dichotomy between what a client needs and what a client wants is a line that isn't always tiptoed gracefully in the strength and conditioning world; the result is often an unhappy relationship between trainer and client. From an aesthetic perspective, achieving a certain physique is dependent on a lifter's body type to start. It may indeed mean spending more time and more training volume on certain regions of the body compared with others. In some cases, it may mean neglecting certain popular exercises while ramping things up in other areas. A body type with very long extremities and a short torso can't be expected to attain upper arm thickness using identical methods and volume prescriptions as a body type with a longer torso and shorter, stockier extremities. Similarly, the effects of a routine with plenty of pressing work on a longer-armed lifter compared with a shorter-armed lifter will be noteworthy and will influence just how to train each body type for more developed chest and shoulder musculature.

The truth is, these are not easy things to just "know" when faced with a new program as a lifter, or when faced with preparing a program for a new client as a coach. This book should serve as your guide for such cases. With no stone unturned, you'll be ready for whatever the training game throws at you. As you can see, a number of psychological, situational, and even cultural and community-based factors can influence training for results. Since the world of weight training can indeed be a bit divisive, it can make for a tougher go when it comes to seeking and finding balance in the quest for proper, healthy, and well-rounded fitness. Lifters often become products of their environment, which can influence the methods they use most. Joining a gym predominately trafficked by powerlifters will likely encourage a lifter to train heavy most frequently in the major compound movements. Joining an Olympic lifting gym may encourage more clean and snatch patterns than otherwise. Belonging to a calisthenics-based studio can mean more bodyweight training and gymnastics work in the program, and so on.

Each of these comes with its own benefits and challenges, including the community peer pressure that can make a lifter think one method or community is better to belong to than the others—which can close one's mind to variety and diversity. A mindset of openness to diversity is necessary to understand and appreciate concepts like the importance of the 11 components of fitness; or variation between goals of strength training, hypertrophy, or conditioning; or even the knowledge that beyond a certain point, attaining more strength yields diminishing returns from a health perspective. This all fits perfectly with the open-mindedness needed to acknowledge that different body types may require different attention depending on the lift and goal in question. And, in truth, why shouldn't they?

Chapter 2

Common Body Types in Sport

Certain body types will prove to be advantageous in certain sports, and as such, individuals with those body types will tend to gravitate toward the sports in which their bodies help them excel.

Tallness is often a desired trait in sports in which a vertical reach is crucial. Tallness helps basketball players reach the 10-foot hoop and defend the basket from other players. In volleyball, tallness helps players strike and block the ball at a greater height. Tallness is valued in American football quarterbacks in order for them to be able to see over the line of scrimmage.

A shorter stature seems to be a better fit for sports in which a lower center of gravity or a lighter body weight is advantageous. In gymnastics, being shorter may mean quicker movements and a better ability to regain balance after aerial feats. Gymnasts are generally very strong for their considerably light body weight, which is important for body control through extreme ranges of motion. Jockeys need to be small and light so their horses can run at optimal speed. Weightlifting can benefit from a shorter height because the weight will have less distance to travel.

Short arms can also be useful for sports like gymnastics—in movements such as the iron cross, in which the body is held aloft between laterally outstretched arms on the rings, shorter levers mean less stress on the shoulders.

Long arms are desirable in sports in which throwing velocity is important. Longer-armed athletes tend to excel at discus and shot put, for instance (Roser 2013). Moreover, leg length relative to torso length can mark a noteworthy difference between stride frequency in sports involving quickness, foot speed, and rate of velocity. Soccer forwards, football running backs, and rugby outside centers all share the same sport demands in needing blistering foot speed with a generally shorter stride length. The shorter the lever (or limb that rests on a pivot point), the faster the potential frequency—and the more advantageous to the sport that demands it.

An overall large frame will benefit, among others, strongman and strongwoman competitors and Highland Games athletes—a bigger, heavier body can generally manage much higher weight and larger, more awkward apparatuses such as stones. In sumo wrestling, it requires a lot more force to move a heavier athlete out of the ring.

In the world of sport, bodies seem to have evolved in the last half century to become more suited (and more exclusive) to the sport in question at elite levels. Compared with the 1980s, female Olympic gymnasts have shrunk in average height from 5 feet, 3 inches to an even more compact 4 foot 9, the wingspans of water polo players have increased, and the heights of NFL running backs and cornerbacks have decreased (Epstein 2013).

Thinking about this trend more deeply, it makes logical sense. At the elite levels of any sport, you will see recurrent examples of an ideal body type that suits the demands of that sport. These physical attributes, coupled with unquestionable skill, are usually what make the difference between an average athlete and a gifted one in the top tier. Despite the fact there are outliers, the world of sport serves as clear evidence that those outliers are eclipsed by the number of athletes who do possess the ideal body type for their sport, or even for their position in their sport. Regardless of sport or body type, the thing in common with all these athletes is they weight train in a gym setting in order to improve their performance. The training is meant to be a vehicle toward getting better at the sport.

But sometimes—intentionally or unintentionally—the training *becomes* the sport. When the focus moves toward weight training as a means to perform in and of itself, or an athlete indeed competes in a barbell-based sport like Olympic weightlifting or powerlifting, similar looks at anthropometry can be very telling. Very few world deadlift leaders possess short arms or torsos relative to the rest of their bodies. Similarly, there are few decorated or internationally recognized Olympic lifters who fit an ectomorph body classification, with long extremities relative to their torso length.

If we zoom the microscope outward to include a greater demographic (not just the elite), we'll find one thing that must remain constant, regardless of the sport: strength training. The ectomorphic basketball player, the short-limbed running back, and the long-armed discus thrower must all find a way to train for strength in the weight room, despite not sharing the body types of gifted strength athletes. That can pose a problem and safety risk for those who aren't informed of how to approach their programming.

Working with a lifter from the general population makes the demand for this individualization that much greater. Being years removed from competitive sport (or never being exposed to it altogether) can mean a less heightened kinesthetic awareness to "make reps work" through athletic adjustments between sets, between reps, or even *within* reps. Uncontrollable factors such as age, prior injury, and skill level (training age) are key players. Not possessing a body type conducive to efficient performance in the weight room forces a general population client to choose exercises, loading, and rep schemes wisely. A personal trainer or a lifter would do well to recognize this, and it's worth deeper consideration. Even a middle-of-the-road trainee—not an athlete, not a competitive lifter—still has goals they'd like to achieve. And that puts them in contest, so to speak, with the weight they're lifting. Anything measurable and trackable with the ultimate goal of progression will mean a prerequisite of sorts of a lifting efficiency that caters most to the thing being measured. Achieving that efficiency—whether it's a squat, a deadlift, an Olympic lift, or a core exercise—will be very much aided by the body type, anthropometry, and leverages of the person performing it.

This idea raises the important truth that the demands on the body can vary depending on the exercise variation in question, and some versions or parts of movements and activities can cater more to a certain body type than another. Taking the example of a 100-meter track and field athlete, we can look at the numbers. Even despite some diversity in the heights of the last 10 Olympic 100-meter male champions (excluding repeat champions) dating back to 1968, with the most common height being 6 foot 2, the shortest champion of the group was 5 foot 9 and the tallest 6 foot 5 (Top End Sports, 2015).

Winning times aside, differences in individual anthropometry can make for differences in how each race is won. Sprinting to max speed is a combination of stride length and stride rate (also known as stride frequency). The ideal situation for an athlete would be to have a correct blend of both of these attributes; too much of one and too little of the other won't equal out to a fast time over 100 meters. Even in a smaller, elite group like the one focused on here, the taller athletes of the group like Carl Lewis, Linford Christie, and Usain Bolt were known for their closing speed despite slower starts, thanks to their stride length. Since a shorter lever equals a faster frequency, the shorter athletes like Maurice Greene were able to achieve maximum speed earlier in the distance by way of a faster start and maintain their top velocity for the duration of the race. The individuals' body types naturally best serviced different parts of the race, with all things equal. Since there was indeed a common height among 100-meter dash champions, it does suggest there is an ideal body type for elite performance, and people who fall out of this range may need to make athletic compensations of some form in order to be in the same category of performance.

Bringing this back to strength training, seeking improved performance—or elite performance—means first examining the lifter's body type to see what movements their anthropometry may be in harmony with in the name of efficiency. Perhaps changes need to be made to the standard version of a popular exercise, or a focus toward higher performance in another discipline within training would be a better option. For example, 5-foot, 9-inch Maurice Greene was a champion 100-meter athlete but wasn't as dominant in the 200 meters, where stride length and speed maintenance are valued more than they are in the 100 meters. Choosing the right focus for an athlete looking to play to their strengths can be paralleled to a trainee looking to get the most out of their efforts in the weight room. It doesn't mean neglecting movements altogether—but it may mean spending less time on some than on others, in the name of improved performance, health, and safety.

Powerlifters focus on three major movements—squats, deadlifts, and bench press. The goal is to move as much weight as humanly possible while achieving the greatest allowable mechanical advantages. A bench-presser with long arms covers a greater pressing distance, which requires more work. The same goes for a tall squatter with long legs or a tall deadlifter with shorter arms (as mentioned earlier). CrossFit applies the "most, most, most" approach with their athletes, using technique that's appropriate for most people, most of the time, under most circumstances. This suggests a goal of facilitating the best performance in the sum of all challenges rather than the most elite individual performance in any one challenge. Despite the generally homogeneous body types found among elite CrossFit competitors, this approach can open the doors to many who may not possess the perfect anthropometry for elite performance in certain gymnastics events but have much more suitable body types for Olympic lifts, running, or swimming. Simply put, certain body types will excel in certain disciplines within CrossFit but may be a bit disadvantaged in others.

For the average person looking to get in shape (or take their good fitness to the next level), it's worth repeating: The sport *is* training. It's beneficial to first decide whether the goal is elite performance to serve an athletic purpose or whether it's all specific to the tasks at hand. Is the goal of a 500-pound (225 kg) deadlift simply for the sake of a 500-pound deadlift or for a healthy spine that doesn't have any problems when the person is running outside or playing a sport for fun? The honest answer to a question like this will influence the decision to pursue the goal.

A scout can look at a young athlete who's tall for his age and determine there's potential for excellence on the basketball or volleyball court. If *training* is the sport, it's similarly wise to first learn whether an athlete has the body type that is suited for it. And a proper place to start would be in figuring out how to determine just what kind of body type the athlete has.

In general, men have tended to be taller than women, and studies have shown that the average height for an American adult male is 5 foot 9 (Fryar 2018). The last five CrossFit Games champions (Mat Fraser, Ben Smith, Rich Froning, Graham Holmberg, and Mikko Salo) are 5 foot 6, 5 foot 9, 5 foot 7, 5 foot 11, and 5 foot 7, respectively. Your athlete might not be going for the next title, but this statistic makes for some food for thought—especially since crowning the champion puts plenty of lifts under the microscope, most of which we will be discussing here. Considering the median height of those five champions falls right into the *average* category, it definitely lends to the idea that average proportions and leverages can service the efficiency and relative ease of compound barbell movements compared with having other physical dimensions. A lifter who's 6 feet tall with a wingspan that surpasses their height would certainly fit the category of being a tall lifter.

In the case of women specifically, their average height is around 5 feet, 5 inches. That will make for far fewer examples of the *tall* category in the absolute form (it's harder to find a 6-foot woman, who would be a tall *person*, compared with a 5-foot-8 woman, who would be tall for the gender). Since 5 foot 8 still fits into average absolute height when referencing weight training efficiency, it's useful to take a closer look at proportions in this particular case. A 5-foot-8 woman with an upper and lower extremity length more in proportion than that of a 6-foot-1 woman would certainly deal with the same challenges and forces as a lifter of the latter height. In truth, the same particulars exist for a 5-foot-8 male with the same proportions. In addition to looking at wingspan relative to total height, one would do well to consider the length of their legs in the same spectrum. From hip bone to foot, if this makes up more than half the lifter's height, they have legs that are fit for someone taller than they are. If these factors exist while also being above 5 foot 10, it's undoubtable that the lifter not only fits the category of being tall but also has leverages that will create the same lifting experience as someone even taller.

Shorter lifters (lifters that fall below the average height by international standards) may not deal with as many issues that plague strength training, thanks to the reduced distance travelled, but they may need to endure other challenges, including having smaller hands and feet or a lighter body weight, which may place constraints on classic strength standards. Which brings up the next point.

The Sport of Training: Strength Standards, Lifting Percentages, and the Body Bias

Even in the world of training for fitness, most people have a goal of becoming stronger as a result of consistent weight training. In the strength training arena, it's common for pundits to apply standards of strength as a metric for lifters to strive for. This may include ideas like considering oneself strong at an elite level when able to perform a 2.5-times body-weight deadlift or a 2-times body-weight squat. First, it's unwise to view strength training, despite all its benefits, as something that's free of risk or disadvantage. We can't act like there's no collateral damage incurred by constantly lifting heavier and heavier weights on a regular basis, or that the joints and connective tissue don't suffer functional drawbacks from dealing with such loads (especially for those who are very strong). If this wasn't a reality, lifters would get stronger and stronger as they aged, with no peak to their performance. Strength training is only part of the picture when it comes to total fitness, and it needs to be approached with a discerning eye. Ignoring other principles of training or indicators that there's indeed a line between a good, healthy pursuit of strength and a less useful one that brings the law of diminishing returns into play can be the start of an injury-riddled downfall for a lifter.

As mentioned in the previous chapter, we're all products of our environments, at least to some degree. And the creators of strength standards couldn't have dreamed up these numbers without having worked with (or been) members of the elite competitor crowd in a given discipline. So, there's some bias there.

In the world of sport, there's direct benefit for football players, powerlifters, Olympic weightlifters, strongmen, and strongwomen to strive for such numbers, but there's a disconnect when we take their strength and try to apply it to Bob from accounting. That, essentially, is the reason most titans of CrossFit are indeed under 6 feet and have average lever lengths. Efficiency of movement is quintessential when you're racing the clock. And if you're not skeletally built for lifting, you're going to have more frustration reaching generic lifting standards. No known strength standard has taken into consideration the size and anthropometry of the individual, and it's time that changed.

Strength standards, training programs, and most fitness recommendations as a whole assume a relatively clean slate, per se, of an injury-free lifter: a blank injury history, an ideal training age, the time per day and week to commit to the demands of the program, and, yes, a body type that's conducive to training this way without any setbacks and with the most linear gains possible. There are not too many exercises that will benefit from having very long legs and arms and a high center of mass. And that's why across lifting-based sports (like CrossFit, Olympic lifting, and powerlifting), that body type doesn't permeate the elite competitors.

Especially when looking at distinctions in size of the individual, it's worthwhile to note the difference between two kinds of strength: absolute strength and relative strength. Absolute strength is very simple to define—the amount of weight a person can lift, by the numbers. In a powerlifting contest, the winner of the contest is the person who possesses the most absolute strength (therefore placing first). Relative strength is measured by a strength-to-mass ratio. Someone who deadlifts 400 pounds (180 kg) at a body weight of 130 pounds (60 kg) will have more relative strength than a person who deadlifts 400 pounds at a body weight of 200 pounds (90 kg). Even though the amount each lifter is moving is the same, the lighter lifter will be moving a weight that's a greater multiple of their body weight.

This is where things get tricky. Following the narrative that a 2.5-times body-weight deadlift is an indicator for strength levels is more useful if the lifter in question fits somewhere in an average spectrum of body types. Notwithstanding proportions, a 180-pound (80 kg) lifter will be more easily found deadlifting 450 pounds (205 kg) (2.5 × 180 lb) than a 280-pound (130 kg) lifter will be found deadlifting 700 pounds (320 kg) (2.5 × 280 lb). A mental shift may be necessary to understand that certain benchmarks may not be as realistic if the body type in question is considered an outlier for elite performance—the same way it's less realistic to assume most 7-foot-tall bodies will be 100-meter Olympic finalists, or most short-armed, stocky builds will be elite football quarterbacks or basketball centers.

This is the grain of salt this book is pulling no punches in providing. Although the content contained in these pages will help lifters of various anthropometries safely improve in their major movements, the caveat that real-world application needs to be kept top of mind—and that it's not useful to play a numbers game with the elite—shouldn't be overlooked.

Remember: perspective. If a member of the general population is looking to improve strength and is frustrated by their progress, it's worth taking a closer look at their programming to see whether they've been force-feeding lifts and trying to place a square peg in a round hole. If you're a coach who creates such programming to the same effect, reviewing the particulars of that programming should be in first order.

Strength Training and Safety: Common Variations in Skeletal Anatomy

Training for body type specificity is useless—even with all the correct pre-scribed exercises—if quality of movement on a basic level is low. Any trainer would do well to do some form of investigative movement testing for a new client, to determine whether each joint has functional integrity and the mobility to move freely through its desired range of motion. Any compensations to achieve simple patterns must be addressed first before loading those patterns. Looking at the skeleton is the first place to start, and it's going to take a few educated guesses since we don't walk around with portable X-ray machines. Even though we can't "see" what's happening, certain tests can allow us to make the most educated of guesses without the use of imaging.

The two load-bearing joints requiring the most range of motion are the shoulder and hip, and both are ball-and-socket joints. Taking a closer look at the hip joint (as seen in figure 1.1 on page 7) demonstrates that some hip sockets are wider set while some are more narrow. Some acetabula have deeper sockets, and others have shallower ones (figure 2.1). Some face more anterior (frontward), whereas others face more inferior (downward).

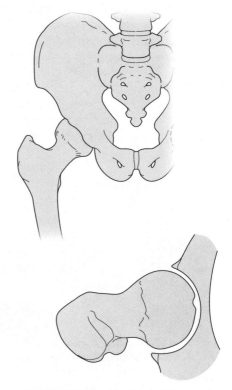

FIGURE 2.1 Hip joint with acetabulum and femoral head.

These particulars can influence a lifter's ease of achieving full hip flexion, especially with various selected stances.

Even a discrepancy of half an inch can make a world of difference on the lifter's performance. If a lifter, for instance, has deep-socketed acetabula that also face inferiorly, the basic squat mechanics suggest the lifter won't be able to achieve a very deep squat without spinal curvature or uncomfortable hip impingement through bottom end ranges. The makeup of the femur—the upper leg bone that fits into the acetabulum to create the hip joint—throws more variables into play. The femoral head should fit nicely into the socket, but the femoral neck—the piece of bone that joins the head to the femur shaft—can be long or short and of various angles relative to the shaft. Because of this, the foot stance chosen as a natural positioning for

Hip Rockback for Testing Range of Motion at the Hip Junction

To test for the correct squatting stance, it's best to look at what range of motion is available at the hip junction, independent of the pelvis and lumbar spine. A quadruped position with the hands, knees, and toes on the floor at about shoulder-width apart is a good starting position. Maintaining a neutral spine, the athlete slowly rocks back toward the heels, with the intention of keeping the spine neutral and simulating a squat pattern while on all fours (figure 2.2). Note at which point in hip flexion the lumbar spine begins to flex, or round. Choose a different foot and knee width, and repeat the test. This time, see whether the curvature happened earlier or later than the time before. Continue repeating the test with varying foot and knee widths, until you find the width that promotes the greatest range of motion with the least (or latest) blockage from the pelvis. This is a good indicator of the foot stance to use when squatting for best results. Coupling this knowledge with the correct mobility drills to groove patterns will significantly help performance.

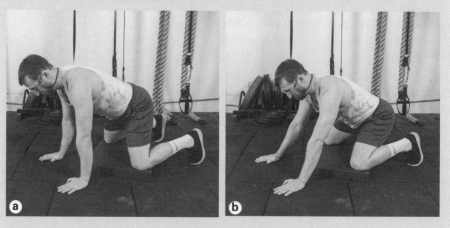

Figure 2.2   Hip rockback: start position *(a)*, and finish *(b)*.

many movements—especially squats and deadlifts—becomes important and case specific.

A lifter whose hip flexion is blocked very early despite trial and error probably doesn't have acetabula conducive to many hip flexion–based exercises. This information can save that lifter a lifetime of training frustrations and chronic pain. It will also allow them to understand that they don't have movement deficiency—they are a prisoner of their own skeleton and must instead move best with what they've been given. That may involve shifting the focus away from a popular movement.

The other major ball-and-socket joint is the shoulder. Of the two joints, the shoulder is the more vulnerable because of its shallower socket, formed by the glenoid fossa of the scapula. In some ways, it's doubly important to possess proper function at this joint, because much of it depends on the strength and movement quality of the structures of the upper back. The shoulder joint is a bit more complex in nature than the hip; healthy movement depends on the thoracic spine and scapula (the midspine and shoulder blade) working properly as the arm moves around (figure 2.3).

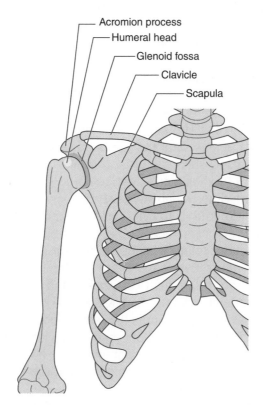

Acromion process
Humeral head
Glenoid fossa
Clavicle
Scapula

FIGURE 2.3　The shoulder joint.

Try this: Have the lifter raise a straight arm over their head (so the biceps are next to the ear) and see what happens to the rest of their body. Does the lumbar spine remain neutral, or does it arch excessively? Does the elbow remain straight or bent when overhead? Can they even place their hand and arm in this position without discomfort or pain? Next, have the lifter reach down and touch their toes with nearly straight knees. They don't have to worry about keeping a flat spine—they can let it round. When they're down there, take a look at their back to see where most of the rounding occurs. Does the back create a smooth hump? Does the lumbar region stay fairly flat while the midback creates a pronounced curvature? All of these differences can have a significant impact on the lifter's shoulder joint and its function.

When there are mobility issues at the shoulder joint, first take a look at the thoracic spine. The thoracic spine is responsible for rotating, flexing, and extending the midback, and for many lifters, this region of the spine presents the most dysfunction in at least one of those actions. When the thoracic spine is limited in how much it can flex or extend, this can "lock up" the shoulder blade, keeping if from moving freely around the rib cage. It's much harder to retract the shoulder blades and raise the rib cage when the spine is stuck in excessive flexion. When this happens, the overhead mobility of the shoulder will be limited, and compensatory actions will be needed if the goal is to get the hand in a specific place in space overhead—in this case, plenty of lumbar spine overarching will make up for lost distance. The result is a false shoulder flexion: The actual shoulder joint is responsible for only a certain amount of flexion until the lumbar spine enters the picture with its extension to help out. This problem would likely be solved by attaining a healthier functioning thoracic spine, especially in its ability to extend. But, similar to the hip joint, other variables may be affecting shoulder mobility that practicing drills will do little to fix. We will further discuss how the spine's curvature can affect exercise in chapter 9 of this book.

The shoulder joint is skeletally made up of four key players: the glenoid fossa, mentioned already, the scapula, the humeral head, and the clavicle. Of course, many tendons, ligaments, muscles, and bursae run through this junction to allow shoulder function. As you can see in figure 2.3, the articulation between the clavicle and scapula (the acromioclavicular joint) deserves special attention because its construction dictates just how much freedom of movement a shoulder will be preprogrammed to have. The bony process of the scapula is known as the acromion and can reliably be classified in one of three designations: flat, curved, or hooked.

A flat acromion process leaves plenty of space for the underlying bursae, tendons, and rotator cuff muscles. When the arm reaches overhead, the amount of space beneath the bone certainly reduces but is still very manageable, making most overhead movements pain free, with all things equal. No modifications or special considerations need to be made for classic movements. Long story short, it's the most optimal shoulder joint construction to have.

A curved acromion leaves a bit less space over the soft tissue structures and as such may require a modification in an overhead pattern that changes from an internally rotated grip to a neutral grip (just as an example). This change rolls the head of the humerus back behind the clavicle to free up some more space and make movements more comfortable and away from impingement risk. The nature of the movement otherwise may not be affected; the lift can still be performed directly overhead, and progressive overload can be pursued using these adjusted parameters.

A beaked or hooked acromion creates more hassle because most overhead work will cause pain and impingement. Even with a modified hand position, a hooked acromion will usually lead to pain or discomfort when pressing directly overhead, often requiring modifications to all (overhead) pressing patterns to change the angle to something more conducive to a smooth, uninterrupted pattern that causes no damage to the joint or tissue surrounding it.

Similar to the hip, of course, there's no way to know an athlete's shoulder classification without imaging done by a practitioner. But this information lets you make an educated guess as to where a lifter fits on the spectrum, and it sheds light on whether or not they're skeletally built for certain types of lifting. Again, there's nothing that can change these structures—it's what people are born with, and they are prisoners of their own skeletons. That means they have to find the modifications, substitutions, erasures, or additions for their programming that make the most sense to promote pain- and risk-free training that still works toward their goals.

Without getting too medical, there are more issues and necessary workarounds than the ones already presented. And when the sport is recreational weight training for fitness and health, and the lifter's "career" span is supposed to be a lifetime, it's necessary to take the needed precautions by first understanding how their body works.

Popular fitness culture will have you believe that pushing through pain, or making adjustments to very commonly used methods of lifting, should be looked down upon as a poor indicator of true performance. In a world of cancel culture, this is a culture that certainly needs to be canceled in and of itself. If an exercise causes pain, it should be stopped. And if trial and error in modifications and technical precision doesn't fix the issue, it may not be something the lifter is doing wrong. It could be the way the lifter's body is constructed, conflicting with the particulars of a certain movement pattern— and an indication to move on to something else. It can be inspirational to see a top-tier athlete training hard and using a mantra of *no excuses, walk in, crawl out* to define their training ideology. As ubiquitous as this mentality is in pro sports, it's equally harmful and shouldn't apply to your client Deborah from finance, the 38-year-old single mother to a 5-year-old child, managing a 45-hour per week desk job.

With this information gained, it's a natural next step to consider the basics of movement as they apply to the most popular patterns and how such movements and patterns are affected by the physical laws of the universe. The truth is, a closer look at the common body types that pervade sports at the elite level should shed some light when we bring things to a personal or client-based level. Even if there are no aspirations to compete, the knowledge that different bodies are constructed differently should greatly influence the choices made on the weight room floor and should highlight that general population lifters are not exempt from this. Their performance in the gym may not be as under the microscope or up for dissection as the performance of an elite lifter or athlete, but factors like anatomical structure can indeed have a serious impact on their limits and whether or not their workouts will be pain free or labored. With this in mind, getting into the technicalities of each movement, in a way, calls for a prerequisite understanding of baseline physical concepts to ease the transition into this subject matter. And that's why we've prepared a little science lesson for you to help you understand how the body works as a biomechanical machine, before diving into the lifts themselves.

Chapter 3

Introduction to Fundamental Movement Patterns

When the term *fundamental* comes up in regard to fitness and training, the first words that typically come to most people's minds are *basic*, *beginning*, and *foundation*. That's a good way to associate the terms, since training that has purpose and is results driven will be contingent upon establishing the rudimentary tenets before getting too advanced.

These movement patterns do just that: establish the fundamentals. They place the greatest emphasis on the physics of movement to help a lifter understand that good biomechanics rely on proper harmonization among several joints, require good mobility, and need every working muscle to contribute to an action. Understanding these patterns means first understanding that training for health and performance relies on focusing on *movements*, not muscles.

On that note, it's worth getting into the details of that distinction. For example, many people think about a common lift and mentally associate that exercise with a target muscle regardless of the size of the movement (e.g., thinking of the bench press as a chest exercise). Similarly, they may think *shoulders* when they see an overhead press pattern. Truth be told, these are definitely the primarily involved muscles for each respective pattern, but the mindset with which the movement is being approached as a whole is very one-dimensional and isolated. The influences of isolation training, physique- and cosmetic-based workouts, and the bodybuilding and fitness competition culture (especially of prior decades) definitely create this mentality.

Alternatively, it's better to understand weight training as a method for loading movements, not just moving loads. This adjustment in mindset brings weight training back to the basics of the original intention: to replicate human movements we do in everyday life, in order to become better, more efficient, and stronger at those patterns. Performing a movement well will help a lifter remain injury free and resilient to any trauma associated with that movement or involved structural complexes.

Movement patterns fall under the following simple categories:

- Hinge
- Squat
- Push
- Pull
- Carry

The carry is the simplest movement pattern, so it isn't discussed separately in this chapter, but the others will be covered in detail later. But before getting into the breakdowns of exercise expectations, it's important to grasp another concept.

Exercise Rules and Principles

Good coaches understand the difference between *rules* and *principles* when it comes to learning, coaching, and cueing exercise. In other words, several fundamentals and basic expectations *must* be in place for a lifter to achieve a safe, high-quality lifting pattern. These are tenets of exercise that every fitness professional should agree upon for the promotion of good health. This encompasses being led by principle. Being led by rules is much more black and white, leaving no room for individual variation based on the case study. Breaking away from this thinking in order to accommodate such diversity is, in truth, the nexus of this entire book. More specific, however, is that one size does not fit all when it comes to "how" to successfully perform a lift. There are many ways to adjust the rules without abandoning the principles.

A useful illustration is a baseball player performing the skills of pitching a baseball or swinging a bat. The principles of throwing a pitch involve generating power from the legs (especially pushing off the rear leg), creating an overhand delivery, and holding the baseball in the fingers instead of the palm. The principles of swinging a bat involve preparing with the legs in order to turn the hips into the swing, using a full rotation of the torso, and keeping the head square and the eyes focused on the baseball all the way through. Certainly, all baseball training coaches would agree on these ideas, while realizing that the arm angle of release will vary between pitchers. So will the comfort level (and decision) between pitching from what's known as "the stretch" and pitching from the windup. Likewise, the individual differences between a batter standing with an open-foot stance or a bunched-foot stance, using a heavier or lighter bat, swinging the bat two-handed or one-handed, or using a high leg kick versus a low one to start the swing are all things that depend on the athlete. All these examples show instances of requirements, being more fluid, all while the principles of execution are being respected. The same can be said of lifting: There is very little one can do but leak strength and power and risk injury when trying to argue with the physical laws of the universe that create an efficient, safe, high-quality lift—and that's what we're exploring in this chapter.

A Closer Look at the Spine

You can think of the spine as the mission control center of every movement pattern. The reason is that the underlying goal of all major lifts, and many major muscles' involvement in those lifts, is to protect the spine and the important role it plays in creating a healthy body. The spine is made up of three regions: the cervical region comprising 7 vertebrae, the thoracic region comprising 12 vertebrae, and the lumbar region comprising 5 vertebrae (figure 3.1). Each region has a different capability and responsibility for rotation, extension, and flexion (both laterally and sagittally).

The spine lives up to being a control center even more so because it encases the spinal cord, which directly communicates with the brain. Nerves that link to and innervate muscle tissue branch out from the spinal cord. In short, all of a lifter's strength, function, and power capacity rely on proper function of the spine. Efficiently performing compound movements is contingent on the spine's remaining in a proper position while under load.

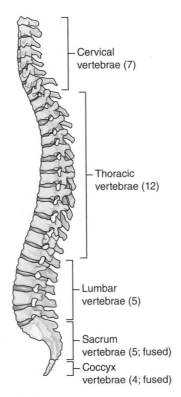

Cervical
vertebrae (7)

Thoracic
vertebrae (12)

Lumbar
vertebrae (5)

Sacrum
vertebrae (5; fused)

Coccyx
vertebrae (4; fused)

FIGURE 3.1   Spine with vertebral groups.

Flexed Versus Neutral Versus Extended

So we're all on the same page, it's best to start by defining each of these spinal positions. A flexed spine refers to the segments of the vertebral column tilting to accommodate a rounded, or forward bending, position. Telling someone to reach down and touch their toes with straight knees will almost always result in a flexed spine—especially through the lumbar region. A neutral spine is the most desirable across most scenarios, where the vertebral column creates basically a straight line, encouraging a very braced core and a well-supported axial skeleton. An extended spine refers to the segments of the vertebral column tilting to accommodate a leaning back, or arching, position. For most people, this is easiest to attain in the lumbar region, especially since the lumbar region has a natural lordotic curve, or arch, to it.

In almost all cases, it's not recommended for a lifter to perform a compound movement with a flexed spine. That doesn't mean the second this happens an injury will be guaranteed—but it does mean the chances have increased. It's an important distinction for an individual to grasp. As a lifter or coach, it's easy to get stuck in the matrix of being a technique stickler who disallows any irregularities in form. Although it may guarantee a client's safety, it might also hinder their abilities to perform what's known as a "grind"—the phenomenon of pushing through a tough repetition and trusting the technique they have worked hard to earn. Time in the profession (and time spent training oneself) can be instrumental in finding a way to strike a balance between the grind and an unsafe movement. Even though this book doesn't encourage overuse of the one-repetition max (1RM) for the general population, the concept of grinding and being closely married to absolutely perfect and flawless technique and positioning is still vital information for people looking for strength gains even in 3M, 5M, or even 8M ranges—specifically because reaching a new rep range max will probably mean a final rep that isn't as clean technically as the first rep of that set.

Neutral

Notwithstanding the preceding information, the ideal for most lifts would be a neutral spine because it promotes the greatest involvement of the musculature on both the front and rear sides of the structure. Remember: The glutes and hamstrings are posterior tilters of the pelvis, since their direction of contraction is downward. The lower abdominals contract upward from the front side of the body, which means when those muscles shorten, they harmonize with the glutes and hamstrings in creating a posterior pelvic tilt. It's only sensible to keep these muscles involved and engaged during loaded exercises because they'll support the lift—whatever it is. With that said, it's important to understand how posterior tilting can act on the spine (figure 3.2).

A typical healthy spine will be softly shaped like the letter *S* when viewed from the side. That means a slight lordosis of the spine (extension) in the lumbar region. Going back to the involvement of the glutes, hamstrings, and lower abs when contracted, posterior pelvic tilting will remove that lumbar extension from the picture and neutralize the spinal position—a terrific starting position for vertical pushes and pulls.

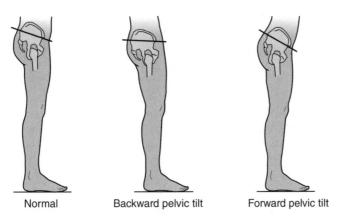

| Normal | Backward pelvic tilt | Forward pelvic tilt |

FIGURE 3.2   Examples of pelvic tilting: normal, backward tilt, and forward tilt.

Bearing load with an overly extended spine can potentiate risk in the same way and isn't ideal when the force angle of the exercise isn't in harmony with said extended spine (more on force angles later). Compression from spinal extension can happen just as easily as compression from spinal flexion, which only further drives home the idea of neutrality being king. In simple terms, compression happens most commonly under vertical loading—namely, standing exercises that involve weight. Bearing load in a standing exercise like a squat, overhead press, or deadlift applies downward stress forces on the spine that can be exacerbated when the spine is not held in a neutral position (i.e., flexed or extended). The discs between the vertebrae are at risk of getting pinched, or impinged, from the loading coupled with the vertebral misalignment, ultimately causing a disc herniation. The compressed region of the spine will pinch the disc and cause it to bulge outward toward the more open side of the vertebra, which results in very distinct pain for the lifter (who at this point would be very fittingly referred to as a *patient*).

Part 1: The Hinge Pattern

Hinge movement patterns, also known as hip-dominant movement patterns, are exactly what their title suggests. The major fulcrum of the movement is the hip joint. The body folds at the hips in order to use the involved muscles to perform the lift. When the hip is the axis of rotation, it places the training onus largely on the muscles of the posterior chain, especially to enforce the previously mentioned neutral spine. The glutes, hamstrings, and erector spinae are three of the most important and prominent muscle groups involved in hinge patterns. The lift variation that naturally comes to mind when thinking about hinge patterns is the deadlift and its variations. It's the quintessential hinge pattern in basically its purest form, and it's a vertical pulling pattern. Here, we'll discuss its requirements in its most basic form: the conventional barbell deadlift.

Barbell Deadlift: Principles of Training

The instruction of the deadlift pattern is as simple as possible, with the shortest list of responsibilities: Stand up with the barbell. The execution, however, can be easier said than done.

In general terms, the setup of a conventional deadlift involves the feet positioned inside (i.e., narrower than) the arms. The hands will grip the bar outside the shins, and the hips will be in a position of greater flexion than the knees. This is the position to assume when preparing to pull a conventional barbell deadlift.

Now, in order for that lift to be performed successfully, more attention to detail is needed. To begin, it's worth noting that the barbell (or other implement) in any vertical pushing or pulling exercise—the deadlift being a vertical pull—needs to travel in a straight line, without any irregularities in its path. The shortest distance between two objects is indeed a straight line, and from a physics standpoint, this means the efficiency of the movement depends first and foremost on respecting this principle. With that physical ruling in mind as a constant, it is the responsibility of the lifter to conform to and support that bar's linear path.

Beginning Stance

The feet should be positioned flat on the ground. They shouldn't roll toward the big toe, nor should the heels start to peel off the ground. The chosen foot width may vary from person to person, but what matters most is that the foot width aligns with the width of the knees and hips. There should be no collapse inward at the knee joint because this will leak power and cause unwanted joint stress on the medial structures of the knee. The bar should be positioned close to the body, since it will finish against the body at the top (and doing so will promote the desired straight-line trajectory), ideally over the midfoot. The hands should be evenly spaced on the bar, just outside the shins. A lifter should avoid a huge gap between the shins and the hands because this will increase pulling distance and hinder the optimal power distribution. To further promote a straight-line trajectory and bar path, the shins should be positioned fairly vertically, relatively perpendicular in angle to the ground, so as not to have the knees or shins impede the bar on its way up the body to the top position.

Spine Position

Most importantly, the spine should be held in a mildly extended position, and this shouldn't be compromised. When someone struggles to achieve an adequate spine position and sets up in a position of flexion, it usually speaks to their lack of flexibility or mobility (or both) and requires addressing. Not addressing this issue means the vertebrae will change position under load, risking injury and breaching the idea of a true hinge-based pattern that uses the hip as the fulcrum. Instead, the spine will need to go into extension as the lifter nears the end of the rep to stand tall, which is not ideal. Similarly, starting out with a neutral spine may be passable and even coached, but think about the effects of the gravity of the weight once the movement begins and the bar starts to leave the ground. Especially if loading is heavy, the immediate result is usually that the spine loses the neutral position and enters flexion (even mild flexion) early in the lift.

An often-forgotten piece of advice that coaches will generally agree on cueing involves neck posture. The cervical vertebrae are part of the spine, and they also need to be positioned neutrally. That means the head doesn't start looking up at the roof—it starts looking down at the floor, slightly ahead of the barbell. This is often referred to as having a "packed neck," and it ensures no cervical extension and no risk to compression of those vertebral discs.

Execution

With the hands on the barbell, the lifter must create tension so that the applied forces are directed to the right places at the right times. It's a general rule of thumb to avoid jerking the weight off the floor; doing so is another way to leak power and lose tightness. The finished product of the setup should be a slightly extended spine with a proud-chested position, while the hands are securely and evenly on the bar. The hips should be distinctly hinged and in a deeper angle than that created at the knee joint, with a head posture that is in alignment. The feet will be flat and in line with the knees, with the toes facing forward (or very slightly outward).

The execution of the movement itself from a biomechanics perspective requires plenty of synchronized action from the muscles of the body. The downward contraction of the hamstrings and glutes is an instrumental component to determine what takes control of the pelvis and works the hardest to initially get the bar off the ground. From the position of greatest hip flexion, the muscles of the lower back have the responsibility of getting tight and braced to create an extended lumbar spine for the setup. If those muscles forfeit that responsibility, the back would be rounded before pulling. The result would be shortening of the hamstrings and glutes to further posterior tilt the pelvis and amplify that technical flaw. Assuming tension and tightness of the lower back in the setup and beginning phases of the pull is the way to have the lower back assume the most control over the pelvis and the pelvic position to prevent unwanted posterior tilting too early in the movement.

As the lift progresses and the bar moves farther from the floor, this control over the pelvis will be handed over, so to speak, to the hamstrings and glutes. The low back musculature will require less work to get out of a flexed spine position because of the torso's angle and degree of hip flexion. The responsibility will be on the glutes and hamstrings to posteriorly tilt the pelvis and stop the lumbar spine from overextending the low back. When lifters fail to do this correctly, you see the overarch and drastic lean back to complete a rep, as opposed to a strong, erect, vertical finish position with the glutes contracted.

As far as the remainder of the upper body goes, the goal of maintaining properly aligned posture with shoulder blades slightly retracted will always be in place. Muscles like the rhomboids and the lower and upper traps work in a generally isometric fashion, but the lats do not, despite popular belief. They shorten because the arm starts at a more shoulder-flexed position relative to the torso at the beginning compared with the end of the lift. The loading in the hands may make it harder for a lifter to conceptualize a loaded shoulder extension, because the force angle in a deadlift isn't directly challenging this action, but this is indeed what occurs.

This indicates a responsibility for tight, engaged lats through both the concentric and eccentric portions of the deadlift, another tricky area where lifters may leak power. Through the ascent, the abdomen should be braced— this means having air in the stomach and a contracted core to help protect the spine and bolster the middle region. The breath should be let out near the top of the rep. The knees and hips should be fully extended for a tall standing position.

Finishing Stance

Lowering the bar back to the floor for the eccentric component of the deadlift basically involves the same steps in reverse. A lifter does well to keep the tension of the lower back, hamstrings, glutes, and lats as the bar travels downward in a straight line. Pushing the hips and buttocks backward while the bar drags itself along the thighs will ensure this trajectory. The shins need to remain vertical so the knees don't impede the bar's path downward. For this reason, it's wise to think about "sitting down" or truly emphasizing a knee bend once the bar has already passed the knee joint on the way down. To be clear, the knees *will* be slightly bent in the first phases of the lowering (on the bar's descent from hip to knee). But they will bend much more, along with a change in shin angle if needed, on the bar's descent from knee to floor.

Hand Grip

The final coaching point to discuss is the hand grip when deadlifting. The most reliably safe grip for the conventional deadlift is a double overhand grip. That means the hands tightly grasp the bar with the palms facing the rear and the knuckles facing away from the body (figure 3.3a). The bar should not be resting in the fingers; rather, it is closer to the palm of the hand, with the thumbs over the fingers and not tucked underneath.

Some lifters (and coaches) encourage the use of a mixed grip—one palm facing away from the body and the other palm facing toward it—when barbell deadlifting (figure 3.3b). This grip will undoubtedly bolster grip strength thanks to the traction being produced on the bar in opposing directions, but aside from increasing the strength of the actual deadlift by the numbers, it doesn't do much to service the body in a healthy way. If you take a look at the injury videos on YouTube, you'll notice that the biceps tendon ruptures some deadlifters unfortunately experience consistently happen to the underhand (palm forward) arm of the mixed grip—never the arm of the overhand palm. The mixed grip essentially asks the body to internally rotate one shoulder while externally rotating the other. It's understandable to conclude that this deliberate imbalance may create or cascade other imbalances through the body, despite a lifter possibly being athletic enough to hide them from plain sight—notwithstanding the benefits this grip may provide for absolute pulling strength.

The mixed grip usually is not coached to a beginner in need of the fundamentals but is more smartly treated as an intermediate tool reserved for heaviest sets. Ingraining a deliberate imbalance or asymmetry when deadlifting, starting with the first warm-up set of the empty bar, is a way to create an injury that's acute in nature or to slowly develop nagging issues of chronic pain.

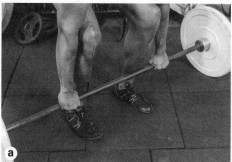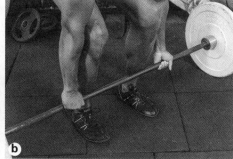

FIGURE 3.3   Barbell deadlift overhand grip *(a)*, and mixed grip *(b)*.

Part 2: The Squat Pattern

At a cursory glance, the squat pattern can be confused with the hinge pattern, but in truth, the two are quite different. Whereas the hinge pattern places an emphasis around the hip as the primary fulcrum, the squat pattern relies on similar starting cues (like a flat-footed position and neutral spine) but also encourages maximal flexion of the knee joint, making the knee the primary fulcrum by comparison. This change shifts the muscular involvement away from being nearly exclusive to the posterior chain. The primary knee extensors are the quadriceps, and their employment in the pattern allows the hips to descend farther than a typical hinge pattern will allow. Another key net result in the change from a hinge pattern to a squat pattern is the difference in tension placed on the hamstring group (Wright, Delong, and Gehlsen 1999). These geometrical changes allow the hamstrings to be less taut, since the origin point of the hamstrings don't have to move as far away from the insertion point to produce the "buttocks back" position. To illustrate: With all things equal, an athlete with a strained hamstring muscle will find it easier to squat down while injured than to hinge over, because of the degree of stretch the latter places that muscle group in compared with the former. This is only augmented by the greater involvement from the quads by comparison to help the pattern.

Barbell Back Squat: Principles of Training

Of the countless squat variations available for consideration, it makes the most sense to view the most popular and most commonly used, instructed, and coached exercise to lay out our groundwork. Irrefutably, that would be the back squat using a barbell as load. This (and any squat) is an example of a vertical pushing pattern; the load is being moved away from the ground thanks to the effort and the force the lifter is placing into the ground with their body. As we already know, loaded movements with vertical orientation require the load to travel in a straight line for optimal efficiency, making a squat pattern fit these criteria. Again, the body must conform to that vertical bar path for a successful lift; what matters is that doing so is accomplished safely.

Beginning Stance

The foot stance for the squat depends largely on individual anatomy. As discussed in chapter 2, finding a foot width that promotes the safest, greatest range of motion is ideal, and that can be achieved through trial and error while using drills like the hip rockback (see page 22) to ascertain individual performance. Fortunately, most coaches have gradually drifted away from a blanket cue for the squat pattern that encourages everyone to select a shoulder-width stance and instead recognize the need for individuality. As such, the cue has commonly become adjusted to "choose the stance that's most comfortable for you."

Moreover, the angle of the feet also needs to be approached on a case by case basis, although it's most commonly coached to keep the feet angled slightly wider at the toes compared with the heels (figure 3.4a). What matters most as a nonnegotiable setup cue is that the knees point in the same direction as the toes—not only in setup but throughout the entire duration of a set as well (figure 3.4b). This can prove difficult if a lifter doesn't have good foot stability or has fallen arches. Alternatively, supporting structures surrounding the knee (such as the adductor group or vastus medialis quadriceps muscle) may need strengthening.

Although placed on the back, the bar needs to be centered over the middle of the foot, dividing it into a front half and back half. Under heavier loads, the body will gravitate toward assuming this spatial position in any case, so as not to stumble backward or pitch forward. This will mean setting up in a starting position of very mild hip flexion; standing vertically will cause the bar to be off-center and probably roll off the back. The Olympic lifting community prefers a bar placement on the back that's higher up on the traps (known as the high bar position); however, the powerlifting community tends to prefer a position lower toward the scapulae and rear deltoids (known as the low bar position). For the purposes of the general population, however, it's most common to select a bar position that rests between the two. When a lifter stands with a proud chest and the shoulder blades pinched together, a muscular "shelf" is created by the trap muscles (figure 3.5), which, when coupled with

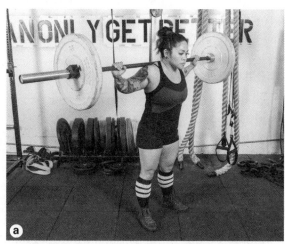

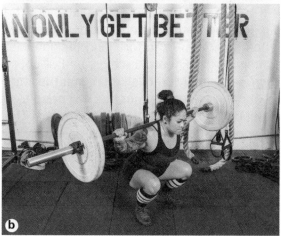

FIGURE 3.4 Back squat: beginning stance (a), and finish position (b).

the hands being placed on the barbell just wider than shoulder width and the elbows raised slightly behind the bar by a few degrees, makes for a comfortable place for the bar to rest.

Speaking of hand placement, a pair of closed fists that create strong (ideally outward emphasized) tension on the barbell helps

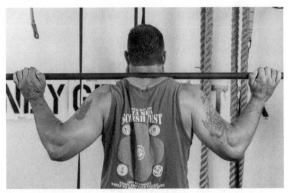

FIGURE 3.5 Upper trap shelf from shoulder blade retraction.

engage the upper back and involve the upper body to make it ready to squat. As in the deadlift, the head position is to be kept neutral. That means it remains in line with the rest of the spine, causing the head and eyes to be facing the floor a few feet ahead of the body.

Execution

Initiating the lift starts on the eccentric rep, by a simultaneous flexion at the knee and hip joints. This allows the body to travel downward rather than hinge too aggressively to face the chest to the floor or knee flex too aggressively to raise the heels and overload the knees and quads. As the body descends, the chest stays up high to maintain a flat spine, and the knees remain open to maintain alignment with the toes (figure 3.4b). This creates space for the hips to travel downward. Ideally, a lifter will possess the mobility for the hips to travel below the level of the knee with the heels remaining flat on the floor and the bar remaining over the middle of the foot in space.

The lowering phase of the squat should be approached with control—not a rapid drop to the bottom position. It's very easy to lose muscular tension when doing this, and forfeiting tension means less support for important joints, like the knees, the hips, and of course, the vertebral segments and sacroiliac joint. Moreover, the faster the lifter descends with the weight, the harder and faster the muscles will need to contract to change the weight's direction and begin the concentric rep. The forces of gravity can make a 135-pound (60 kg) bar (for example) feel like a lot more than 135 pounds. Through the descent, the abdomen should be braced—this means having air in the stomach and a contracted core to help protect the spine and bolster the middle region. Pressing the feet into the floor while intending to remain as upright as possible with the upper body is the key to getting "out of the hole"—or returning to standing position from the bottom phase of the squat.

It helps to squeeze the glutes and focus on maintaining alignment between the knees and toes. The breath should be let out near the top of the rep. The squat finishes in a nearly standing position, with fully extended knees and near fully extended hips.

A simultaneous knee and hip flexion causes the buttocks to "sit back" slightly as the movement progresses. The idea of sitting in a chair is a common analogy used to help lifters understand the emphasis and mechanics. As you'll learn, differences in anthropometry will dictate just what cues work for what people, and individual anatomy plays its role in determining what biomechanics will lead to a successful lift.

Spine Position

Many coaches will warn against the phenomenon of "butt wink" at the bottom of a squat, where deeper depths (or even sometimes shallower depths, depending on the lifter's mobility) elicit a pelvic "tucking," making for a posterior pelvic tilt as the lift approaches the bottom. There is a distinction to be made, however. The lumbar spine can be in one of three positions at the bottom of a squat—or during any other movement, for that matter: extension, neutral, or flexion (figure 3.6).

Carrying a heavy load—or even a relatively light one—with the lumbar spine in flexion is unquestionably dangerous. However, many form sticklers and fitness pundits start cringing the moment they see *any* change in spinal position at the bottom of the squat. Their hearts are usually in the right place, but it's easy to cry "flexion" when the truth is closer to neutral.

As learned in the deadlift section, bearing a load with a neutral spine is safe and actually ideal, and it doesn't negatively affect strength. And some degree of butt wink is necessary to come out of back extension and into a

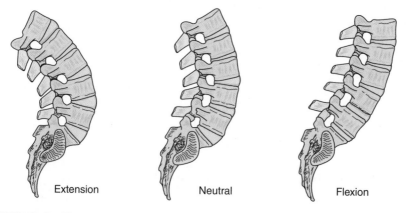

       Extension   Neutral   Flexion

FIGURE 3.6   Three types of lumbar curvatures: extension, neutral, and flexion.

neutral position. Lifters who don't know this often stop the lift short, claiming they're protecting their lumbar spine, even though they're only slipping into neutral and forfeiting plenty of available range of motion below parallel. Because of the setup requirements of a back squat, seeing some butt wink is to be expected, since the spine begins in a slightly extended position for most people who perform it. For a real-life example, look at any Olympic lifter, or any of the strongest athletes who use full-depth squats, and you'll see their back will slip into a neutral spine position at the bottom. It's important to recognize this as acceptable. When the back slips into a position of flexion, however, this spells trouble for the lower back and its segments.

When it comes to squatting, an optimal way to approach squats for the fewest potential problems is to achieve access to as much depth as possible. This gives the lifter the power of choice as to what depth is needed for a given workout. If all these particulars can be respected, it makes for a good start.

Part 3: The Push Pattern

Pushing (or pressing) can be done at an almost unlimited number of angles, first and foremost because it requires the engagement of the shoulder joint. The shoulder is a ball-and-socket joint, and thanks to its structure, it is the most mobile joint in the body. However, the extreme mobility of the shoulder and the complexity of the joint, plus the fact that we tend to use our arms for just about everything we do in life, means the shoulder is at a high risk of injury (Quillen, Wuchner, and Hatch 2004).

Pressing movements are compound movements, recruiting the shoulders, chest, and triceps to work in unison to complete the press. The stability and strength of the wrists are also challenged in most pressing movements. Pressing often requires a fair amount of work from other areas of the body—the lower body is of great importance in the push press and the jerk, for instance.

Pressing movements can strengthen the shoulder complex at the angle of the press, but, of course, proper form is key in order to minimize injury risk. Training the shoulder at multiple angles is extremely beneficial to keep the shoulder complex strong, stable, and less likely to be injured. For the purposes of this book, we discuss the bench press as a horizontal push and the military press as a vertical push.

Bench Press: Principles of Training

The bench press is often seen as the epitome of gym strength. We've all heard the all-too-familiar question: "Hey, how much can you bench?" While it's up for debate as to what the pinnacle of the demonstration of strength might be, it is fair to say the bench press is an extremely effective way to overload the muscles of the chest, contributing significantly to strength and hypertrophy of the upper body.

There are many nuances in the execution of this seemingly simple movement. There is, for instance, much controversy about whether a bench press should be performed with an arched spine, as is fairly ubiquitous among powerlifters (figure 3.7*a*) or a flat back, as is commonly seen in the form of bodybuilders (figure 3.7*b*).

There is little conclusive evidence regarding the advantage of an arched-back bench press over a flat-back bench press, and few studies have examined the differences between these variations. One study saw no change in one-repetition max (1RM) between the two methods (Garcia-Ramos et al. 2021). Another noted that an arched-back bench press lent itself to about 11 percent less vertical displacement in the press and about a 20 percent shorter barbell to glenohumeral moment arm (Pinto and Dickerson 2021).

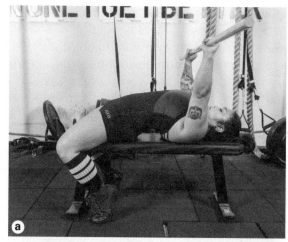

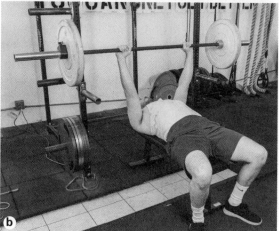

FIGURE 3.7 Bench press with arched back *(a)*, and flat back *(b)*.

One feature of the arched-back bench press is that it shortens the path of the bar since the height of the lifter's chest is much greater than in a flat-back bench press. This can lead to the ability to press a significantly greater weight than from a flat-back position (although not necessarily, if the results from the Garcia-Ramos study hold true). This may be a great advantage in competition or for purposes of lifting the most weight possible. The lifter, however, will mainly gain strength within the range of motion that the bar is pressed. For strength increases in a larger range of motion, a smaller arch or a flat-back bench press might be preferable.

A moderate spinal arch in which the shoulders are retracted ("pulling the shoulder blades into the back pockets") will create a more stable support base from which to press. This also helps prevent anterior rotation of the shoulder and helps recruit the latissimus dorsi, allowing for a stronger, safer lift. It is important that the athlete not overly pinch the shoulder blades together. The shoulders should be pulled down the spine as much as possible, angled slightly toward each other.

A common view in coaching the bench press is that the movement starts from the feet. In other words, implementing leg drive—shoving the feet into the ground as the bar is pressed from the chest—is important for an optimal lift. Leg drive is another element of bench pressing that does not have much research behind it. One study on the subject found that five weeks of training recreationally active college-aged men in the leg-drive bench press was about the same as training a standard bench press in increasing 1RM (Gardner et al. 2021). The authors of the study conclude that the athlete should decide which method works best for them (which, honestly, is fairly good advice for most movements).

A few rules do hold true in the bench press. To maximize efficiency, the bar should travel in the straightest vertical line possible when it is pressed. This, as we see in chapter 4, is the shortest distance from the bottom of the press to the top of the press, resulting in less time in transit for the bar (and therefore the least amount of effort for the lifter). That said, the shoulder joint does not really lend itself to a completely vertical bar path. The bench press path will generally follow a slight J shape—it will travel backward a bit before pressing straight up. The lifter will ideally position the bar over the shoulder joint as quickly as possible by the end of the press. It is surprisingly easy to misjudge the end point of the barbell—many lifters end up with the bar somewhere over the face or the abdominals. It can help to have a focus point—something to aim the bar for—during the press. This can be as simple as the coach's hand during a training session.

Beginning Stance

The bar should always touch somewhere along the chest at the bottom of the bench press. A common instruction is to aim the barbell for the xyphoid process, although some lifters prefer to press from midchest at the nipple line, and others prefer a different touch point. The touch point will vary based on the lifter's levers, degree of arch, and grip width, and it may take some experimentation to discover the optimal touch point for a particular lifter. Regardless of location preference, the bar should not bounce off the touch point in the lift. The barbell should also not sink into the chest—it simply stops there momentarily before being pressed.

Execution

Whether the athlete is flat-backed or arched, there should always be three points of contact with the bench for the duration of the bench press. The buttocks, upper back, and head should not be raised at any point while the bar is unracked and in the hands of the lifter. Some powerlifting federations allow the head to come up in the bench press, but many do not; it's best for the lifter to understand the rules of their particular federation should they intend to compete.

The wrists should ideally be as straight as possible for the duration of the lift. Some lifters choose to wear wrist wraps to help keep their wrists in a more vertical position. Ideally, the forearm of the lifter will also remain as vertical as possible, so that the final arm position creates a perpendicular line to the ceiling.

The width of the hands in a bench press is an individual choice, depending on where the lifter feels strongest and safest. Powerlifters often use the widest grip legally allowed in order to reduce the length of the path of the bar and thus potentially maximize the amount of weight lifted. For most lifters, a grip slightly wider than shoulder width should provide some of the load benefits of a wider grip while keeping the shoulders in a relatively stable, comfortable position.

Clearly, many factors in the bench press can be manipulated to optimize the lift for a particular lifter and a particular purpose. If the lift feels stable, safe, and strong, the average lifter has likely found a formula that works for them. A good coach can help tweak these variables in order to produce the best results for that lifter's goals.

Military Press: Principles of Training

The overhead press is an important exercise for building strength, mass, and power in the upper body. Overhead press movements are common for Olympic lifters and strongman athletes, but many types of athletes can benefit from pressing a weight overhead. The implement used (dumbbells vs. barbells vs. logs and so forth) depends on the goals of the athlete, and different implements can certainly be accessory exercises for the target equipment. We focus on the barbell military press since it is often the method used in competition and because more weight can generally be pressed using a barbell—dumbbell presses tend to be less stable, and the barbell can allow the stronger arm to take over the lift to some degree to accommodate a heavier load. That said, dumbbell presses can be an excellent accessory movement for the barbell military press, in part because the weaker arm cannot rely on the dominant arm to help complete the press. Thus, the combination of managing a heavier load using a barbell and strengthening the nondominant side using dumbbells can be the ultimate one-two punch for optimizing strength in the overhead press.

There are multiple ways to get a weight overhead.

- In the strict press, the lower body is not used to assist the press—the athlete simply presses the bar to lockout from the upper chest.
- The push press is generally used for a weight that is too heavy for the lifter to lock out without any assistance. In the push press, the athlete dips several inches at the knee while the body remains upright, then forcefully drives back upward with the legs until they are straight again

(as in a jump without leaving the ground) in order to create momentum that helps push the barbell off the chest and toward lockout.

- The jerk can be used for a weight that is too heavy to be push-pressed. In this movement, the lifter initiates the press with an extremely powerful dip and drive. Once the barbell is airborne, the athlete dips a second time, placing themselves under the bar and locking out there rather than pressing the bar overhead. The jerk can be done with a split leg position or a parallel position, but either way, the feet should be placed parallel to each other by the end of the lift. The jerk requires a tremendous amount of athleticism, stabilization, and coordination to execute successfully, but it is an excellent method of getting a very large amount of weight overhead, should that be the goal.

The military press can also be done from a seated position, either on a bench (also known as a seated military press) or on the floor with legs splayed out in front of the lifter (also known as a Z press). These movements remove leg and torso drive completely, thus putting the onus of the press fully onto the upper body.

We discuss the strict standing press in this book.

Beginning Stance

To perform the standing military press, the athlete grasps the barbell with an overhand grip at the appropriate width for their levers. Ideally, the barbell will sit at the base of the hand so it is as close to directly over the bones of the forearm as possible. The bar should remain over the midfoot as much as the athlete is able. In this way, the barbell will be over the line of force for a strong, efficient press. Ensure, too, that the thumbs are wrapped around the bar—while a thumbless grip is possible, there is a much higher chance of the bar rolling out of the athlete's hands without the thumb around the bar.

Ideally, the bar will start around the athlete's collarbone, depending on the athlete's flexibility. The muscles of the abdominals and upper back should be contracted so that the torso feels tight and locked in place, and the elbows should be directly underneath the wrists and as perpendicular to the floor as possible. Too wide or too narrow of a grip will prevent a vertical forearm, so ensure that the chosen grip width allows for vertical forearm placement. The athlete may lean back slightly from the hips. The key word here is *slightly*—the lifter should not lean back so far as to turn the movement into a sort of incline chest press.

Execution

The athlete presses the bar toward the ceiling and, at the same time, force-fully straightens the hips to generate a bit of momentum to help drive the bar up. The bar should travel in the straightest line possible. Many lifters will try to loop the barbell around the face—this is an inefficient pathway that will detract from the power behind the press. The lifter should aim for the nose (they will not hit it), and the elbows may flare slightly in order to best support the bar as it travels upward.

Finishing Stance

As the arms lock out at the top, the athlete should push their head between their arms so that the bar is in line with their ears (or slightly behind the ears, depending on flexibility). The athlete should be in a tight, upright position in which as many muscles as possible are contracted to create the most stable base of support beneath the barbell. Lowering the barbell in a controlled manner back to the racked position completes the repetition.

There is no one-size-fits-all direction for the width of the stance or the width of the grip on the barbell for a military press, so the lifter can choose what feels best. However, a slightly wider than hip-width stance could provide a more stable base of support for the press, and many lifters find a slightly wider than shoulder-width grip on the bar to be a comfortable and effective position from which to press.

Part 4: The Pull Pattern

Much like the push pattern, pulls can be done at any number of angles thanks to the versatile structure of the shoulder joint. In a pulling exercise, the athlete is either pulling an object toward their body or pulling their body toward an object. A pull horizontal to the body is generally a form of row, while a vertical pull is known as either a pull-up or a chin-up, depending on the position of the hands. That said, it is possible to change the angle of the pull by adjusting the athlete's body position or arm so that the pull tracks in a diagonal line with the body.

While the main movers in the push movements are the triceps, pectorals, and anterior and medial deltoids, the main movers in the pull movements are the biceps, latissimus dorsi and other muscles of the back, and deltoids (mainly posterior). Pulling movements like rows and pull-ups are also effective for strengthening grip and can engage the abdominal muscles to varying degrees. We discuss the pull-up as an example of a vertical pull and the seated row as an example of a horizontal pull.

Pull-Ups: Principles of Training

For many people, the pull-up is an important test of upper body strength. This exercise has been used in physical fitness tests for many military branches worldwide as well as for law enforcement and firefighters. Pull-ups can be performed just about anywhere a bar or sturdy ledge is available.

The premise of the pull-up is very simple: Grasp the bar with a neutral parallel grip or another desired grip (if the palms face the lifter, the movement is a chin-up). Starting from a dead hang, pull the body toward the bar until the chin is above the bar. Lower until the arms are straight, and repeat as desired. As with all lifts, however, there are many nuances to the pull-up.

Kipping Pull-Up

The popularity of CrossFit has made the kipping pull-up a subject of debate—does a kipped pull-up count? Clearly, a kip provides a great deal of momentum to drive the athlete over the bar. The answer really comes down to what the athlete wishes to achieve in the pull-up. According to one study, the kipping pull-up recruits a great deal more of the lower body and torso than do strict pull-ups (DiNunzio et al. 2018; Williamson and Price 2021). However, the biceps brachii and latissimus dorsi are significantly more active in the strict pull-up as opposed to the kipping pull-up. Therefore, if the goal is to simply get the chin over the bar as many times as possible, or to do a motion that recruits more of the lower body, the kipping pull-up would likely be the better option. If the goal is to use the pull-up as an upper body strengthening exercise, the strict pull-up is superior to the kipping pull-up. For our purposes, we discuss the strict pull-up only.

Hand Grip

Another point of contention about the pull-up is the grip position—is neutral grip superior to parallel grip, or is another grip more effective for building upper body strength? According to a study by Dickie and colleagues (2017), when a parallel-grip pull-up was compared against a neutral-grip pull-up, a chin-up, and a pull-up done on two ropes, all grips had similar effects on muscle activation in the biceps, brachioradialis, middle deltoid, upper pectoralis major, lower trapezius, latissimus dorsi, and infraspinatus. However, the parallel-grip pull-up demonstrated significantly more activation in the middle trapezius than the other grips tested. Depending on the athlete's goals, this may be a point to consider when selecting a grip for the pull-up.

Proper Form

There is no full consensus on the absolute proper form for a pull-up. For some, the movement is simply "grab the bar, pull the chin up over the bar, lower." For others, the shoulder blades should be "packed" (i.e., depressed) and the body should be in a gymnastics hollow position for the duration of the movement. There does not seem to be much research on which method is best. The hands, as well, are not necessarily required to be wrapped around the bar, with the thumb over the fingers. Athletes might choose a hook grip, a thumbless grip, or another grip that suits their particular preferences and needs.

Because the form for the pull-up is not entirely standardized, the athlete should simply perform the method they prefer. There are, however, two nonnegotiable elements in the pull-up: It must begin from a dead hang position (arms completely straight at the elbow) and must finish with the chin over the bar. Everything else depends on what makes the most sense for the athlete's goals, preferences, and, of course, levers.

Seated Row: Principles of Training

The seated row is not designed to be a 1RM lift. Because the muscles of the back are involved in maintaining posture, they tend to respond well to high-repetition movements. Therefore, the seated row is an excellent high-volume exercise for hypertrophy in the posterior chain. It has been found to be particularly effective for the middle trapezius and rhomboid muscle groups in comparison with pull-down exercises (Lehman et al., 2004).

Although the seated row can certainly be performed with a static torso, the amount of weight the lifter can pull is limited by the amount of weight that can be pulled by the arms. While beginning lifters can benefit from a stationary torso pull in the process of learning the mechanics of the lift, more advanced lifters may have more hypertrophic or strength-based goals, necessitating the use of far more challenging weights. In this case, the lift becomes more dynamic: The torso becomes more active in the movement in order to provide the momentum needed for more weight to be lifted.

Beginning Stance

The lifter positions themselves with their feet braced and hands gripping the handle of choice. The seated row allows for the use of a variety of handles. The lifter should choose a handle that makes sense for the goals of the lift (a competitive rower, for instance, might want to choose handles that place the arms in a position that mimic the sport). For the purposes of this book, we concentrate on a neutral shoulder-width grip.

Execution

Keeping the spine as straight as possible, the lifter rocks forward from the hips, creating a stretch in the hamstrings and the muscles of the back. As the lifter pulls the handle toward their torso, they drive powerfully back from the hips while keeping the spine straight, so that the motion of the torso adds to the power of the lift. In the final position, the lifter's torso will be at a slight backward angle (up to about 45 degrees), elbows pulled as back and toward each other as possible, shoulders depressed and "out of the lifter's ears."

Again, there is no standard hand position for the seated row. There are many variations of this exercise, some of which require the torso to be braced and in which the rocking back and forth motion would not be applicable. There is some benefit to be gained from programming different types of horizontal row patterns, depending on the goals and specific needs of the lifter.

Understanding the cues of basic patterns in their conventional intended execution is no doubt a stepping stone to becoming a good personal trainer, strength coach, or trainee. Just like learning the big lifts can provide a lifter with knowledge to set the foundation for true strength and muscle development (and allow for a rite of passage to get more specific with training goals and exercise selection after the fact), learning these lifts in their most standard form can help one understand the physical requirements of the lift itself, before getting into particulars about leverages, joint angles, and body types. For this reason, we found this to be a very fitting place to start and the smoothest transition into deeper physics of movement—plenty of which you'll read about in the following chapter—so deeper terminology can be simplified by finding a bridge to the real-world application of a weight room–based example. The great news about the fundamental patterns is this: Their requirements will never change. It will always be a game of efficiency against the laws of the universe, and the better someone understands this, the faster their rate of change as a lifter—or as a coach to lifters.

Chapter 4

Levers and Forces

The lengths and proportions of our body levers can limit our ability to maintain textbook form when performing any athletic activity. That's why certain body types seem to gravitate toward certain sports—the proportions of their levers may be optimal for certain types of movement. One obvious example is that tall, long-limbed athletes tend to make better basketball and volleyball players. That doesn't mean short-limbed athletes can't excel at these sports, but it does mean they need to find ways to compensate for what they lack in limb length. A shorter basketball player may, for instance, be better at dribbling and at maneuvering around other players more quickly, so training those specific skills can work to their advantage. Finding ways to increase jump height and throwing power and accuracy will also benefit shorter players, since they are naturally farther away from the basket than their taller counterparts.

In this chapter, we discuss the role of levers and forces in the body—essentially, the physics of the human body. While studying physics topics can feel complex, dry, and "mathy," it can help you understand how unique bodies respond under loads. That can give you a roadmap to manage body levers so they perform optimally, which leads to better performance and lower risk of injury. If you have a basic understanding of these concepts and apply them appropriately, you can use them to your advantage (and your athletes' advantage) in the weight room and in competition.

Forces

To discuss levers, we must first define *force*. The dictionary definition, taken right from *Merriam-Webster*, is "strength or energy exerted or brought to bear: cause of motion or change : active power" (Merriam-Webster 2021).

In simple terms, force is an action taken on an object in order to move it or change it. Force must have both size and direction. A force can be a push or a pull, and it can be active (e.g., lifting a weight) or reactive (e.g., stopping a boulder from rolling down a hill). So you can apply force to, say, a lump of clay to turn it into a vase, or you can apply force to a barbell to snatch it overhead.

Forces can be balanced or unbalanced. Balanced forces mean the forces acting on the object are equal to the forces resisting them. In other words, the object receiving the balanced forces will not move, because neither force is greater than the other. Forces need to be unbalanced to create motion. If one force is greater than the opposing force, movement or change will occur. So if an athlete puts 200 pounds (90 kg) of force on a 150-pound (80 kg) weight, that weight will move in the direction the athlete is pulling or pushing it.

Gravity

There are vertical forces acting on an object at any given time. The vertical forces that push downward are gravitational forces. The vertical forces that push upward are ground reaction forces—the forces that act from the ground in opposition to the downward force of the object in contact with the ground. In a stationary object, the ground forces will be equal to the weight of the load in contact with the ground. So for a deadlift, for instance, the ground will exert a force upward equal to the weight of the athlete and the bar. Ground forces will change depending on the type, speed, and direction of the movement of the load.

There will always be both an active and reactive force on a given object—if an athlete is lifting a barbell, they are applying active force. Gravity, however, is trying to push that barbell back down to the ground and is supplying the reactive force. You could also say, if you like, that gravity is the active force, trying to push the weight to the ground, and the athlete is the reactive force, trying to pull against gravity, because Newton's second law does not specify which force is the active one. Either way, two forces are always applied.

From a mathematical perspective,

$$\text{Force} = \text{mass} \times \text{acceleration}$$

This means that when force is applied to a particular object, it will move at a proportional speed in the direction of the force applied. When we're applying this to sport or strength training, the muscles apply the force, and the object could be anything from a weight to the body itself (as in sprinting or calisthenics or simple postural mechanics). The other type of force involved in strength sports is gravity. Weight training is, at its base, the ability to overcome a gravitational pull (e.g., a heavy weight).

The acceleration of the object to be moved will increase either with a greater force (i.e., stronger, more powerful muscles that are able to produce great effort) or a smaller mass (i.e., it is easier to move a 3-pound [1.5 kg] weight with great speed than a 300-pound [135 kg] weight).

Friction

Friction is a force that occurs when one surface slides across another, like a sneaker across a floor. If the bottom of the sneaker has good tread on it, the friction will be higher than it would for a sneaker with a worn-out sole. If the floor is made of smooth, freshly waxed linoleum, there will be much less friction than there would be if the floor were made of rubber tiles. Friction can prevent a runner from slipping and sliding or can make a weight sled a lot harder to pull across a surface. This force is affected by the smoothness of the materials sliding against each other, by the shape of the sliding surfaces, and by the forces acting on the surfaces in question, among other factors.

Friction doesn't play much of a role in the lifting of free weights, but in the case of machine-based training, it can be important. In a cable machine with sliding plates, for instance, or on a Smith machine, the amount of friction on the weights and cables can add to the total weight being lifted (Cotterman, Darby, and Skelly 2005).

Air Resistance

Air resistance is exactly what it sounds like—the force of air on an object moving through it. Air resistance will be most apparent in airborne sports— throwing a projectile, jumping, leaping, diving, cycling, and so forth. It is affected by the speed of travel of the projectile, how big the traveling object is, and the shape and surface of a body (an aerodynamic object is designed to travel through the air with minimal air resistance). Some machines use air resistance instead of weights for training, but in weightlifting, air resistance tends not to come into play much.

Axial Forces

Axial forces are the sum of all the forces that act directly on the center axis of an object. These forces can be shear forces or compression forces. In the case of the human body, such forces will generally act on the joint, and they have the potential to change the joint structure for better or for worse. The forces on the joints increase joint stress and strain. Understanding how these forces affect the human body is imperative for both improving performance and minimizing the risk of injury.

Shear Forces

Shear forces push part of an object in one direction and another part of the object in the opposite direction (figure 4.1). A deadlift with a flexed spine will create much higher shear forces across the spinal discs than will a deadlift with a rigid spine. Deadlifting with the bar farther away from the body will also increase shear forces on the spine, as will deadlifting with a more upright trunk. (Escamilla et al. 2001).

Increasing these shear forces isn't necessarily a guarantee of injury (which is why it isn't uncommon to see elite lifters intentionally perform deadlifts with a rounded spine and have no major aftereffects), but it can increase the risk significantly. Understanding the degree of shear on an athlete's joints during a specific movement can be a valuable tool in weighing the costs and benefits of movement technique. In a squat, for instance, factors that can increase joint shear include a deeper squat, a narrower stance, a faster speed, a forward torso lean, and bouncing at the bottom of the squat (Bengtsson, Berglung, and Aasa 2018). A decision must always be made as to whether an increase of shear force in a lift is worth the increased risk of injury.

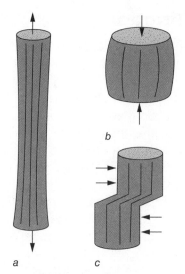

FIGURE 4.1   Example of tension *(a)*, compression *(b)*, and shear *(c)* forces on muscle.

Compression Forces

Compression forces push or pull the ends of an object inward toward each other, causing an object to become more compact. The bar in a bench press, for instance, puts compressive forces on the joints of the wrist and elbow of the lifter. Changing the width of the hands in a bench press will change the way these compressive forces affect the lifter's joints (Chou et al. 2008). This may provide a useful method for rehabilitating injury in an athlete or for adjusting the lift so it produces minimal pain in a joint.

Tension Forces

Tension forces pull the ends of an object away from each other, creating a stretching effect. If you think about a game of tug-of-war, the athletes are creating tension forces on the rope. In a deadlift, the weight of the bar will create tension forces on the arms of the lifter, pulling at the wrists, elbows, and shoulders. There is a very common concept in lifting called time under tension, which simply means the amount of time the body spends in a lift with a force creating tension on the muscles. In that deadlift, the time under tension would be the time it takes to get from the bottom of the lift to the completion of the lift. It can also describe lifting volume—how much time the muscles spend under tension for the duration of a working set.

Tension can also refer to tightening the muscles under a weight in order to keep the body upright and feeling solid at the start of a lift. A lifter will create tension in their body, for instance, when walking out of the rack for a squat with a barbell on their back. The lifter might "brace for a punch," lock the legs, squeeze the glutes, and pull the elbows and hands close to each other in order to create tension in the upper body. Without appropriate tension, the lifter will simply collapse under the bar.

Levers

The body is a simple machine, meaning something that can transmit or modify force in order to perform work (i.e., move an object). Much like a crane lifting steel girders or a pair of tweezers pulling out a splinter, the human body can be seen as a system of levers. The forces we put on those levers stress our bodies in different ways, and those stresses can lead to results such as muscle hypertrophy, strength increases, or even injury.

Characteristics of Levers

All levers have two basic parts:

1. *The fulcrum, which is the pivot point of a lever.* In the human body, the fulcrum will generally be a joint. In a biceps curl, the fulcrum is the elbow. In a squat, there are multiple fulcrums—the knee, the hip, and the ankle. The more complex the lift, the more levers come into play. When multiple levers are working together, they increase the leverage that can be produced. This is why a lifter can generally move a lot more weight in a squat, which uses multiple fulcrums, than in a biceps curl, which uses only one.

2. *A rigid arm that connects to the fulcrum in some capacity.* The arm should not break or bend, or else the lever won't work very well. In the human body, the arm will likely be a bone or series of bones. In a leg extension, the arm is the shin, or more technically, the tibia and fibula. In a deadlift, the arm is the collective bones and joints of the spine, held together as a unit by the contracting spinal muscles.

The load is the object that is to be moved (for the purposes of this book, a barbell, dumbbell, or other type of weight), and the force is what is applied to the lever to move the load (i.e., muscle action).

Mechanical advantage defines how effectively the application of a force on a simple machine will move an object. The mechanical advantage of a lever system can be determined by the following equation:

Mechanical advantage = length of effort arm/length of resistance arm

The higher this ratio, the better the mechanical advantage. A mechanical advantage of 4, for instance, means it would take one quarter of the effort to lift the load than if you were to do it without a lever.

So, the farther a load is from the fulcrum, the more effort it will take to move that load. This is why you will generally need much lighter weights to do straight-arm exercises such as a lateral raise than bent-arm exercises such as a biceps curl. It is also why it may be more challenging for an athlete with longer arms to perform a lateral raise with the same weight as an athlete with shorter arms.

While a load farther away from the fulcrum will take more effort to move, that load will also move faster and for a longer distance than will a load that is closer to the fulcrum. When speed is the goal, a lower mechanical advantage would generally be desirable. It is for this reason that a longer-armed person might be a better thrower than someone with short arms. The longer the distance of the object to be thrown (the load) from the shoulder and elbow (which would be the fulcrums in this case), the faster the travel over a longer range for the object.

Classes of Levers

There are three basic classes of levers.

First-Class Levers

First-class levers are set up like a seesaw, with the fulcrum between the effort and the load. This is the least common type of lever in the human body. The head is an excellent example of a first-class lever, where the fulcrum is the atlantooccipital joint, the load is the anterior portion of the skull, and the force is applied by the muscles that extend the neck (figure 4.2).

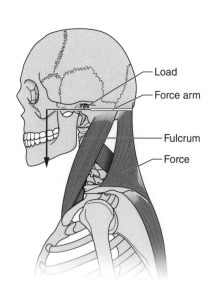

There aren't very many first-class lever exercises in the weight room. The most obvious example would be neck extensions. There are a few others, though. A triceps extension or dip is a good example

FIGURE 4.2 Example of fulcrum, load, and force on head and neck.

of a first-class lever exercise—the elbow, as the fulcrum, would lie between the load (the weight) and the effort (the triceps).

Second-Class Levers

In a second-class lever, the load is between the effort and the fulcrum. A wheelbarrow is the most common example of this type of lever—the fulcrum is the wheel, the load is whatever is inside the wheelbarrow, and the effort is the handles of the wheelbarrow. The mechanical advantage will always be greater than 1, because the effort arm will always be farther from the fulcrum than the load arm. Second-class levers always produce more force but at the expense of range of motion and speed.

One example of a second-class lever in the human body is a calf raise. In this case, the ball of the foot is the fulcrum, the load is all the load-bearing forces of the body plus whatever weight is being used, and the effort is applied to the heel of the foot by the calf muscles.

A push-up is a kind of second-class lever, but in this case, the lever itself (i.e., the body) is the load, which makes it an interesting example (figure 4.3). The fulcrum is at the toes (or knees, depending on how the push-up is being done), and the effort is the hands pushing into the floor. A push-up from the knees has a shorter distance to the fulcrum than a push-up from the toes, so less of a load is shifted to the hands and less effort is required to execute the movement.

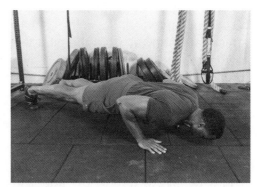

FIGURE 4.3 Example of push-up as a second-class lever.

Third-Class Levers

Third-class levers are the most common type of lever in the body. The load is on one end of the lever arm, the fulcrum is on the other, and the effort is between the two. In a third-class lever, the load arm will always be longer than the effort arm, so the mechanical advantage will always be less than 1. This is great for increasing the speed and the distance the load travels, but not as much effort will be produced. A low mechanical advantage means low efficiency—third-class levers are therefore the most inefficient type of lever. The load will always be farther from the fulcrum, so we need to generate more force in order to move those loads.

There are many examples of third-class levers in the human body. A biceps curl is a very simple example of a third-class lever (figure 4.4). The biceps brachii attaches to the tubercle of the radius and the deep fascia of the forearm. In the biceps curl, the

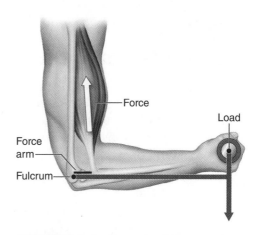

FIGURE 4.4 Example of biceps curl as a third-class lever.

elbow is the fulcrum, and the load is whatever is on the opposite side of the biceps attachment point (e.g., a dumbbell, barbell, wrist weight, band).

As you can see, knowing the attachment points of muscles is very useful for determining the location of the force within the human body. One formula to determine effort in a third-class lever is as follows:

$$\text{Effort} = \text{load} \times (\text{distance from fulcrum to load/distance from fulcrum to effort})$$

This means that the farther the force is from the fulcrum, the easier it will be to move the load. So, in the case of the biceps curl, if the biceps were to attach farther away from the elbow joint, it wouldn't need to work as hard to lift the load in question. Similarly, if the load were in the middle of the forearm, it would be far easier to curl the weight.

Newton's Laws

Newton's laws explain the relationship between the movement of objects and how they respond to the forces acting on them. They're just the beginning of what we now know about these relationships, but they're a very important place to start.

Newton's First Law of Motion (Law of Inertia)

The law of inertia states that an object in motion will keep moving unless an external force acts on it. So if an athlete is pulling a barbell off the ground, it will keep flying up unless gravity pushes it the other way.

Similarly, an object at rest will remain at rest unless a stronger external force acts on it. If the barbell is too heavy for the athlete to lift, it won't move. The athlete must therefore exert a force greater than the weight of the barbell in order to make it move.

Newton's Second Law of Motion

Newton's second law states that the greater the force applied to an object, the more that object will accelerate. The object will accelerate proportionally to the amount of force applied and will move in the direction of the force applied. It will also move inversely proportionally to the mass of the object. This law can be described as

$$\text{Force} = \text{mass} \times \text{acceleration}$$

which we discussed earlier in this chapter.

If we want to look at that equation a different way, we can see it as:

$$\text{Acceleration} = \text{force/mass}$$

From this perspective, the acceleration would be lower for a larger mass with the same force applied. You can imagine trying to run pulling a wagon versus trying to run pulling a truck. The truck is going to move a whole lot slower for the same amount of force. If an athlete performs a barbell clean, they are producing a great deal of momentum in order to accelerate the bar into the racked position. However, if that athlete produces more momentum than they are able to properly control and decelerate, that barbell could continue to accelerate and potentially cause a lot of damage.

Newton's Third Law of Motion

Newton's third law of motion states that for every action, there is an equal and opposite reaction. We touched on this earlier in the chapter, when we discussed active and reactive forces. If an athlete tries to deadlift that barbell on solid ground, the ground will push back on their feet and keep them from sinking into the earth. But if that athlete tries to deadlift that same barbell in quicksand, the ground won't be able to generate the equal force to keep them above ground, and they will end up at the bottom of the quicksand pit. Similarly, if an athlete pushes a weight sled across the floor, friction will push back against the sled to try to keep the athlete from pushing it forward. What makes the sled move is the athlete's ability to push harder than friction is able to push back.

Angular Motion

When we discuss angular motion, we are talking about movement around a fixed point. This movement is due to any force outside its center of mass. One example of angular motion is a windmill—the wind pushes the blades of the windmill outside their axis, and the blades turn as a result. In the human body, angular motion simply describes the movement of a limb around a joint, which accounts for any movement in the human body, from sitting up to walking to lifting.

Torque

Torque is the rotational force that causes a lever arm to turn around an axis. If your body is going to do any kind of movement at all, it needs to generate torque. Torque determines how much force a muscle will need to produce in any exercise, so it is a very important concept to understand when discussing the human body in motion.

You'll see torque applied in the weight room within different coaching cues: in the bench press, for instance, a lifter might be told to "bend the bar" as they try to press it. This application of torque causes the shoulders and arms to rotate into a more stable position for a stronger bench press. When an athlete is instructed to "push their knees out," torque is used to rotate the hips and knees into a stronger squatting position. In a push-up, an athlete might be cued to "screw their hands into the floor," which rotates the elbows and shoulders into a more stable position for pushing.

Torque is dependent on three factors: the amount of force applied, the angle of the force applied, and the length of the moment arm. These are all variables that can be manipulated in the gym and in sport in order to improve movement efficiency and power.

Line of Force

The line of force is the direction in which an object is being pulled or pushed. Gravity is always pulling straight down, so that line of force is easy to measure. The line of force of a punch, on the other hand, is in the direction of the punch.

Moment Arm

The moment arm is the perpendicular distance between the line of force and the axis of rotation (in the case of the human body, this would be the joint). The bigger the moment arm, the greater the angular force. The greatest amount of torque is produced at a 90-degree angle. The smaller the angle, the closer your bones will be together, and the more stable the structure will be.

This explains why a biceps curl, for instance, is most challenging when the elbow reaches the 90-degree angle and becomes easier beyond that. At 90 degrees, the biceps need to produce the most force to move the weight (see figure 4.5).

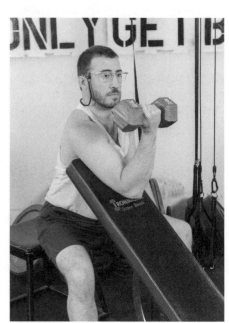

FIGURE 4.5 Example of biceps curl as force versus moment arm.

Angular Velocity

Angular velocity describes how fast an object turns around its axis and is calculated in radians per second. A *radian* is a measurement of the ratio between the circumference of a circle and the length of the radius of the circle. Angular velocity has both magnitude (in this case, a speed measured in radians) and a direction of travel. One example of angular velocity is the arm of a pitcher in baseball—how fast the ball in the hand is moving about the shoulder and elbow. In a squat, the angular velocity is dependent on how long it takes the lifter to reach the bottom of the movement.

An interesting study that demonstrates the relationship between torque, lever lengths, and angular velocity in sport comes from Fleisig and colleagues (1999). In this study, the authors compared the pitching kinematics of younger baseball pitchers with older, elite pitchers. The authors found that all the pitchers had very similar arm speeds. However, the more experienced pitchers had longer arms and more muscle mass. The older pitchers needed to produce more torque in order to create the same speed in a bigger, longer arm, and the combination of the higher torque and longer, bigger limbs meant the baseball was thrown at a much higher velocity.

A skater with their arms pulled in would have a much higher angular velocity than a skater with their arms extended, and a diver with limbs pulled close to the body would have a much higher angular velocity than a diver with extended limbs. One way angular velocity can be calculated is by this equation:

Angular velocity = angular displacement (radians)/time (seconds)

In other words, the shorter the time taken to travel from one point to another, the higher the angular velocity. In a squat, one might measure the angular velocity taking place at the ankle joint, the knee joint, and the hip joint—how quickly the bones travel toward and away from each other in each of those locations. A higher angular velocity in this particular movement may have a sport-specific benefit but might also lead to a higher risk of injury (Schoenfeld 2010), so it is a factor worth examining.

Angular Distance Versus Angular Displacement

Angular distance is a measure of how far an object moves around its axis. Angular displacement, however, is the distance between the starting and finishing points of the moving object. The angular distance of a hammer in track and field would be the circular path the hammer moved, while its angular displacement would simply be the straight line between where the hammer started moving and stopped moving. The angular distance at the elbow in a bench press would be the change in the joint angle between the bottom of the press and the top of the press. The angular displacement of that same bench press would be the angle formed between the initiation of the press and the final position of the press.

Moment of Inertia

The moment of inertia is a body's resistance to rotation or movement. Mass is a major determinant of the moment of inertia—the greater the mass, the easier it is for that body to resist changes in motion. Consider a 100-pound (45 kg) person trying to use their body to stop a truck that is slowly rolling forward—that truck would be able to resist stopping pretty easily. The distribution of mass is also a factor in the moment of inertia. A figure skater, for instance, will spin faster when they bring their arms toward the center of their body, thus reducing the moment of inertia. If the skater extends their arms or puts them up overhead, the skater will spin more slowly, and the moment of inertia will be increased.

The moment of inertia provides a value to the effort it would take to change the speed of a rotating object—starting the rotation, stopping the rotation, speeding the rotation up, or slowing it down. One formula that can calculate the moment of inertia is as follows:

$$\text{Moment of inertia} = \text{mass} \times \text{distance from axis}$$

The higher the moment of inertia, the more force is needed to change the object's rotation. An increase in mass or an increase in distance from the axis can increase the moment of inertia. An object can potentially have multiple moments of inertia, so this equation only touches the surface. A diver, for instance, will change the location of different segments of their body in order to increase the speed of a midair twist, turn, or somersault and changes them again in order to land in the water gracefully. Each body segment has moments of inertia that need to be considered in order for the dive to be ideal.

Linear Versus Angular Momentum

Linear momentum is the linear movement of any moving mass. It is the product of an object's mass and its velocity:

$$\text{Linear momentum} = \text{mass} \times \text{velocity}$$

An object with larger mass or speed will have a higher linear momentum. A huge athlete running at full speed, for instance, will be harder to stop than a smaller, lighter, slower athlete. Similarly, it will be far easier for an athlete to decelerate a 2-pound (1 kg) weight than it would be to decelerate a 50-pound (20 kg) weight.

Angular momentum is the relationship of angular velocity to inertia. In essence, the angular momentum is the movement of a spinning object. One way it can be calculated is as follows:

$$\text{Angular momentum} = \text{angular velocity} \times \text{moment of inertia}$$

In a long jump, for instance, angular momentum comes from the trunk, arms, legs, and head working together in order to both prevent rotation and maximize the distance of the body moving forward in space. The angular momentum of each moving part contributes to the angular momentum of the body as a whole. A high angular velocity or a high moment of inertia will increase the angular momentum.

The law of conservation of angular momentum states that if there is no force or torque applied to an object, its momentum will not change. This is very similar to Newton's first law, which states that an object in motion will remain in motion unless an external force is applied.

Impulse

Impulse is the amount of force produced within a short amount of time. In other words, it is the amount of force and time required to change the momentum of a mass. The more time spent applying force, the more the momentum will change.

Impulse is generally calculated in Newtons per second. A Newton is a measure of the force it would take to move a 1-kilogram mass 1 meter per second squared. Impulse can be calculated as:

$$\text{Impulse} = \text{force} \times \text{time}$$

Impulse is often discussed in Olympic weightlifting, throwing, resistance training, sprinting, jumping, and other movements requiring the generation of a lot of force in a short amount of time.

The subject of forces and levers can be complicated and confusing. It is also a vast area of study with far more detail than is covered in this chapter. However, it can be extremely useful to have at least a cursory knowledge of this information. Movement is, in essence, physics. Having a basic understanding of the concepts covered in this chapter can help you see how the segments of the human body work together to produce movement, and how the configurations and proportions of those body segments might be manipulated to produce the greatest advantage for a particular lift or action.

PART II

Exercise Optimization

In order to properly understand the lift adjustments based on body type, it's important to first know the variations that exist. Of course, the human body can come in all shapes and sizes, but we've narrowed things down to 13 commonly seen physical descriptors.

Tall

Men, on average, are taller than women. The average height of the male across major continents (as mentioned in the introductory chapter) is 5 feet, 10 inches, while the median height for women is 5 feet, 5 inches. This means 5 feet, 10 inches would normally be considered tall for a woman but right on average for a man. Since our mentions of body type relate to leverage as applied to resistance training, it's fitting to keep things consistent to one metric for height of a lifter, regardless of sex. Therefore, for clarity, any individual above 6 feet should be considered tall.

Short

Similar to the tall category, the distinction between males and females based around average height needs to be considered. The same height that would normally be considered average for a woman would be considered short for a man. For our purposes, anyone under 5 feet, 4 inches should be considered short.

Big All Over

This is independent of a lifter's height and has more to do with mass. A man or woman fitting into plus-size clothing (size XL and above for men, sizes 12 and above for women) would be in this category. Larger than average individuals may need to make special considerations for various exercises to respect the amount of space they occupy.

Short Arms and Long Legs

The combination of short arms and long legs is a slightly less common variation, but it can definitely have an impact on both upper and lower body patterns.

Short Legs and Long Arms

The individual who can nearly scratch his or her kneecaps while standing upright can definitely find movements they may gravitate toward. Having a big wingspan means a greater range of motion in various upper body movements. However, some movements may be more difficult to perform well or more difficult to do safely.

Long Torso

When the distance between the hips and the top of the shoulders takes up more than half of the body's height, this can require key modifications for movement patterns. Depending on the lift, having a long torso can affect the low back and knees.

Long Torso, Short Legs, and Long Arms

Now we begin getting into subcategory specifics. This body type is less frequently seen, but it can be found in the sporting world and in fringe aspects of competitive lifting.

Long Torso, Long Legs, and Short Arms

When an overall tall body height is combined with a high center of gravity and a short reach, this can mean a giant range of motion for some lifts and a short range for others.

Short Torso, Short Legs, and Long Arms

This body type is basically the opposite. The dimensions here would make for a shorter overall height and a big wingspan and would likely reverse the demands of the preceding category.

Short Torso, Long Legs, and Short Arms

Carrying the majority of one's mass in the lower body means more than just considering geometry when squatting. There's a definite carryover to other lifts and how their volume can affect parts of the upper body. That includes the spine.

Long Femurs and Short Shins or Long Shins and Short Femurs

The relationship between the upper thigh (femur) and the tibia (shin bone) can largely affect the angles and rate of joint change relative to the other joints of the body when performing a big lift. This relationship can have a serious impact for specific mobility demands of the lower body.

Small Hands

This category is fairly obvious in that hand size will directly affect movement patterns in which an implement is held in the hand or a lift that requires grip strength.

In the lifting chapters that follow, don't expect 13 body type breakdowns for each movement pattern. There will not, for example, be a subsection on leg length in the overhead pressing portion since lower limb variety has little to no impact on overhead pressing strength and efficiency. Instead, the part II chapters will mention only the body types most affected by the lift in question and any body type category that has any mechanical pertinence in the execution of the lift.

Chapter 5

The Deadlift Pattern

The deadlift follows a vertical pulling pattern that is a hip-dominant movement. That makes the hip the major axis around which the rest of the body travels to promote a straight-line bar path when the lift is in action. We've already spoken about the basic techniques for the lift in its conventional setting in chapter 3, and in chapter 1 we briefly touched on certain areas that could make a deadlift more of a challenge to some lifters. With that said, let's look at what can promote a high ceiling of performance for deadlifts and work from there.

The Perfect Conventional Deadlift Body Type

As far as strength is concerned, the first thing to consider is the pulling distance between the floor and the barbell when in the lifter's hands. The less, the better. With that said, a lifter who has longer arms will be in a better natural starting point than a lifter who has very short arms (figure 5.1). A quick look into the elite competitive world of powerlifters with great deadlift numbers will confirm this.

The second natural aid to the conventional deadlift pattern is just how much the lifter's legs can contribute to the lift. Of course, the deadlift largely depends on the lower body, but because the knee angle is far from 90 degrees for most people who perform it, the lower body involvement is very biased toward the hamstrings and glutes. By extension, the lumbar spine will deal with more forces under loading compared with a truly knee-dominant pattern like squats. Because of this, the proper torso angle can go a long way. The hips should be positioned at a lower starting point than the shoulders. When the hips (and glutes) are kept lower, the knees can bend to a greater degree when setting up for the pull. Greater knee bend potentiates greater quadriceps contribution and more leg drive. Assuming the lifter has the correct spine position and no lumbar flexion, the likely result will be a strong pull that spares the lumbar spine of the unwanted burden of handling most of the loading—potentially in an undesirable position. This lends to the idea that a longer torso with average-length legs would be best suited for barbell deadlifting while respecting fundamental mechanics and allowing the movement to remain hip dominant as a whole.

Last but not least, it's common sense that an athlete can lift only as much as they can hold. With that said, a lifter with larger hands will have a much easier time gripping a barbell, delaying their need to settle for a mixed grip or the use of aids like lifting straps. Larger hands will cover more surface area of the bar's circumference so it won't slide out of the hand when pulling. You also need to remember what was discussed in chapter 1 regarding pelvic anatomy. Setting the feet up so that they, the

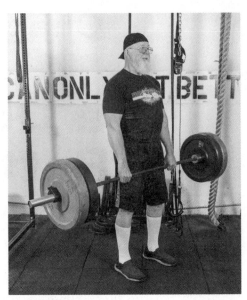

FIGURE 5.1   Deadlift finish position for a lifter with long arms.

knees, and the femurs are in corresponding alignment with the hip sockets might mean a wider stance for someone who is wider built. Since the hands belong outside the shins in a conventional deadlift, this can result in a much wider than ideal hand position on the bar for clearance, creating a greater pulling distance (and more potential for a rounded spine in the start position).

In summary, a lifter with a long torso, long arms, and large hands will be well suited for conventional barbell deadlifting. But that body type doesn't describe everyone. And people who don't fit this category need to know the right variations and coaching cues to suit their body types.

Lifting With Gear: Lifting Belts and Hand Straps

Gear, referring to equipment or accessories designed to improve the safety or performance capacity of a given lift, is something many lifters swear by, or swear against. There are many polarized points of view when it comes to wearing gear of any sort when lifting. Our advice tends to stay right down the middle.

To be clear, the purpose of a lifting belt is to create an additional brace to stabilize and protect the lumbar spine (figure 5.2). Belts are to be worn tightly and uncomfortably; they are not a fashion accessory or piece of clothing that a lifter wears through the entire workout—only during individual sets. The lifter applies force with the core against the lifting belt, using their abdominals and air pressure during the hardest part of the lift (the bottom phase, where the hips are in greatest flexion). Successfully doing this can stabilize vulnerable areas of the lift and contribute to a strong pull. If you see someone at your gym wearing a belt loosely, or never taking the belt off between sets or even between exercises, know that the item is being misused.

If a lifter has a history of injury to a key area—in this case, the lumbar spine—then we recommend wearing a belt properly when deadlifting, especially if the plan is to lift heavy. It's one thing to expose the muscles and discs

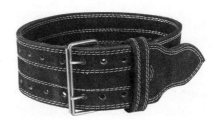

FIGURE 5.2   Lifting belt.
artisteer/iStockphoto/Getty Images

of the lumbar region to stress with the intent of making the region stronger and rehabbing it from prior injury (and preventing a reinjury), but we don't believe the time to push those limits should be during an actual deadlift training session. Train beltless using other exercises to push those thresholds.

As far as hand straps go, they serve two purposes that may compete with a lifter's goals, depending on what they are. Wearing straps will increase the amount of weight an athlete can potentially lift, since the lifter's own grip strength is now being aided by a firm, tightly wound strap that contributes to the pulling tension and force. If a lifter wants to build more true strength in the most natural form possible, there may be some benefit to being exposed to heavier than normal weight, but the lifter won't be holding that weight all on their own, which means less muscular and neural connection attached to the effort. Alternatively, for hypertrophy purposes, if a lifter is trying to take their grip out of the equation and place a greater emphasis on muscles of the posterior chain for development, wearing hand straps is a way to achieve this. Straps can prove especially useful when deadlifts are performed for higher reps; they allow for added volume without the grip fatigue that can frustrate a lifter's efforts.

Deadlifting: Short Torso and Long Legs; Tall

These body type variations are among the most common to experience difficulties when deadlifting. The arm length can be short, average, or long in classification; in each case, the majority of the problem ends up coming in the form of starting geometry. Since the legs are longer than the torso, the center of gravity is higher and the axis point (the hip, where the body is meant to hinge) is farther away from the floor and not in a perfect place for a balanced recruitment of all the major muscles of the lower body. Most lifters who have this body type display one of two compensatory patterns when pulling the barbell:

1. They round the lower back during execution because of insufficient flexibility or mobility.

2. The bar travels around the knee instead of straight up, breaching the efficiency of a vertical path and leaking energy and strength.

Lifters with this body type require higher hips to maintain a relatively vertical shin angle (which will prevent the second issue). The by-product of this change in hip position, however, is less quad involvement and more posterior chain involvement—similar to the positions assumed in a Romanian deadlift. Greater dorsiflexion is required to employ the quadriceps, simply because of leg length. That adjustment gets in the way of ideal lifting physics for this variation of the movement.

Rollaway Setup Method for Tall and Long-Legged Lifters

First and foremost, ensuring a good back position can pose problems for tall, long-legged lifters. The lifter may be allowing their hamstrings to maintain control of the pelvis for the entire duration of the lift, and that's not ideal.

As mentioned in chapter 3, in a typical deadlift setup, assuming a flat lumbar spine while bent over in a pulling position gives the lower back musculature the most control over the pelvis, allowing it to slightly anteriorly tilt in preparation for the pull—creating the mildly arched lumbar spine that's desired. As the lift progresses, the glutes and hamstrings contribute to extend the hips. Their contraction will give them a growing amount of control over the pelvis and gradually posteriorly tilt it as the movement nears completion. It's important to respect this trade-off, so to speak, so the right muscles win their part of the power struggle at the right time.

A good way to achieve a flat lumbar spine is to assume a full squat position with a rounded back before setting up to pull (figure 5.3a). This allows the hamstrings to stay relaxed and not pulled taut, and the lifter can pull *up* into the starting position rather than reach *down* for it (figure 5.3b). That all gives the lumbar spine a much better chance of achieving the neutrality or slight extension necessary for a safe, technically sound pull.

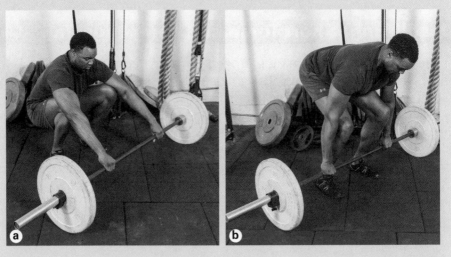

Figure 5.3   Deadlift rollaway method for tall lifters: start position *(a)*, and end position *(b)*.

Best Variation: Trap Bar Deadlift

Using a trap bar for deadlifting can go a long way in fixing the problems for this body type variation, primarily since there is no longer a bar blocking the shins from traveling forward. This allows for a deeper seat position, which can make the back angle better resemble the ideal geometry for a conventional deadlift. Since the weight surrounds the lifter rather than being in front of the lifter, the path of the load can still travel vertically upward without any penalty of being dorsiflexed with an angled shin, and the quads have a chance to better contribute (figure 5.4). This adjustment in geometry means lower amounts of stress on the lumbar spine when compared with the conventional deadlift using a barbell (Swinton et al. 2011).

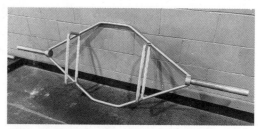

FIGURE 5.4   Trap bar.

The trap bar allows the lifter to pull with a neutral grip from one of two positions: high handle and low handle. Depending on the make and model of the trap bar, the difference between handle heights can be anywhere from 4 to 8 inches (10-20 cm). If the lifter has adequate mobility, using the low handle setting (by flipping the trap bar over before loading and lifting) can rival the range of motion created by a barbell deadlift from the floor, while providing the additional benefits that this particular body type requires for success.

Similarly, the width of the pulling handles can vary from bar to bar. Some handles are narrower in distance at 20 inches (50 cm), whereas others can be up to 25 inches (65 cm) apart. Keeping these things in mind can affect your strength and performance training, especially if the numbers and percentages matter for tracking purposes.

If using a trap bar, the lifter can apply just as much training volume as an ideal deadlifter would. There's no need to reduce the amount of time spent pulling if the lifter's body is in an ideal environment that will be friendly to the joints. With all things equal, they can safely and effectively use high-volume methods. We'll go into more detail about overall deadlift training volume later in this chapter.

If All You Have Is a Barbell: Four Modifications to Barbell Deadlifts

It's a definite reality that the trap bar may not be an easily accessible piece of equipment for many lifters looking to use it. If the gym you're in doesn't have one, it's important to know how to manipulate barbell deadlifts to receive similar benefits. These four variations to the conventional barbell deadlift can go a long way.

Deadlift From Blocks

Simply using plates, low step platforms, or blocks to elevate the pulling start point is a great introductory hack for lifters who lack the mobility or body type to excel at conventional barbell deadlifts from the floor (figure 5.5a-b). No one said there is a rule that the floor must be the actual floor. A lifter can still receive all the benefits deadlifting has to offer, in a range of motion that's best suited for their height or leg or arm length. Especially if the plan is to lift in the lower rep range for heavier percentages, this can allow a lifter to do so with far less risk.

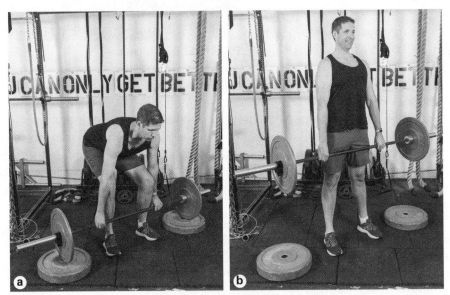

FIGURE 5.5   Deadlift from blocks: start position *(a)*, and finish *(b)*.

To deadlift from blocks, all conventional deadlifting cues remain the same. The only difference comes in the form of the position of the bar relative to the ground—which creates a slight advantage for a lifter with a tall height or long legs and a short torso and arms.

Paused Deadlift

Essential in anyone's lifting journey is the practice of making lighter weight feel heavier in the training effect it delivers—and this will be achieved based on how the reps are performed. Adding a distinct pause a few inches off the ground on the way up forces the spine to remain neutral and prevents the hips from shooting upward first. Likewise, the quads and glutes get a better chance to contribute to the lift thanks to the added time under tension, making the lower back receive the assistance it needs and deserves. This lift won't be performed with a typical working weight; the load will need to be reduced by around 20 percent for the same rep ranges, and that's a good thing. It means the lifter can still train hard and feel taxed, while dealing with less absolute loading that may encourage risk under normal circumstances.

Paused deadlifts can do wonders in addressing spinal position, and they can also help with balance. There should be a slight backward emphasis (about 5 degrees) when picking up the bar to counterbalance the load in front, especially when it's heavy. Being completely vertical at the top of a deadlift probably means the lifter let their back dominate the lift and forfeited some hip drive. Finishing up on a backward slant of about 5 degrees properly counters the load.

Remember, this isn't a trap bar that distributes the weight evenly around the body. It's a barbell, and all the weight is in front. Using the paused deadlift can help the lifter sit back ever so slightly in order to stop the torso from lurching forward and throwing off the force curve.

Isometric Deadlift

The good thing about using an isometric deadlift is that the lifter can create maximum force at every segment of the lift, which is something that cannot be duplicated as long as the bar is in motion and the person is capable of actually lifting it. Applying force against an immovable object makes up for a range of motion that a lifter would typically pass through only using conventional deadlifting methods.

There are a number of ways to use this technique with the deadlift, depending on the setup of the gym. Most commonly, setting up an empty bar in a squat cage, with the pins situated at shin level above the bar instead of below it, is a useful approach. The lifter sets up as they normally would and pulls the bar hard up into the pins (figure 5.6), attempting to lift the entire squat cage off the ground (assuming they cannot). Have the lifer hold for sets of 10 to 15 seconds, using 60-second breaks. Then move the pins up to a higher level and repeat. Do this at every segment of the deadlift in order to strengthen the entire movement piece by piece.

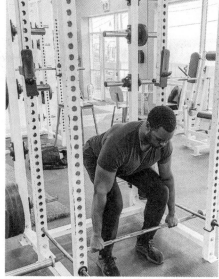

FIGURE 5.6 Isometric deadlift in squat cage.

If you don't have a squat cage that can accommodate this idea, simply load a barbell on the ground to 150 percent of the lifter's 1RM, or a weight you're certain they can't budge—and do the same thing. Load that heavy barbell on some blocks or steps for a higher pulling position and repeat. Then use higher blocks or steps, and so on. Isometrics drastically reduce the risk for injury while allowing the nervous system to exert itself at basically full force. Since the body isn't changing position while applying force, the window for harm is much smaller, and isometrics thus prove themselves to be a terrific supplement for tall or long-legged lifters looking for safe ways to add strength to a conventional deadlift. Sharing the total weekly volume between conventional isotonic deadlift work and isometric deadlift work is a wise call to optimize the risk–reward ratio.

Eccentric-Free Deadlifts

There are different pulling styles when it comes to deadlifting, and two of the most common are the touch-and-go method and the dead-stop method. Touch and go requires the bar to glance off the ground briefly, and under control, between reps. That means plenty of control in the lowering phase and added time under tension for the lumbar spine. In a perfect world, this would lend to more strengthening of the lumbar region—but if someone is not ideally built for deadlifting, too much time under tension may not be the best, especially if they're stuck with a barbell and pulling fairly heavy. In such cases using a dead-stop method (where the bar is lowered fairly quickly to its starting position and allowed to settle on the ground for one or two seconds between reps) can be the best bet. Focusing instead on eccentric-based movements that don't involve such high loads can be a difference maker.

Deadlifting: Big All Over; Long Femurs (Short Shins); Long Shins (Short Femurs)

Something that larger, wider, heavier lifters and lifters with a discrepancy between femur and shin length have in common is that in order to have a successful barbell deadlift, they need proper clearance of the bar; they do this by creating space for their bodies to sit as comfortably as possible in the starting position. It isn't as simple a task as it sounds. Whereas big lifters or lifters with femur and shin discrepancies may get along well with the trap bar—just like the lifters in the previous section—it's important to note that this set of categories does not take a lifter's height into consideration. In other words, the lifter could be 5 foot 4 but still be large, heavy, and wide or have the limb specifics listed here. A high-handle trap bar deadlift may be a potential solution, but it will create a very short range of motion that may not lend itself to training time under tension and a full range of motion.

Because the goal is a relatively balanced contribution from all the muscles involved while sparing the lower back of rounding or added (unwanted) loading, it's worthwhile to understand the compensation patterns that are likely to happen when all things are equal.

A bigger lifter likely won't be able to achieve the same degree of hip flexion as a smaller (or leaner) lifter would, because of the amount of mass they carry around the hip region and midsection. That mass will block the leg's ability to move closer to the torso and achieve greater hip flexion. For this reason, the lifter will be stuck in compromise by way of letting the lumbar spine round to reach the barbell. The problem may not be solved by elevating the bar either. The hip sockets and their placement on the pelvis were briefly touched on in chapter 1. On that note, when considering people with wider frames, it wouldn't be a stretch to imagine they have a wider distance between acetabula. A quick way to determine natural foot placement for a conventional deadlift is to see where the feet gravitate toward being placed during a vertical jump (or a short series of vertical jumps for a more accurate inference). The feet will tend to stay hip-width apart, resting under the hip sockets, which can make for a wider than normal conventional deadlift stance when viewed from the naked eye. This allows for better clearance for the torso to reach down without as much rounding, but it may present a new issue because the hands will need to be placed even wider than the already wide legs. This may exceed the limits of the lifter's flexibility and mobility. There's an answer for this, but first, let's consider the lifter with long shins or long femurs as a parallel.

In both cases (long femurs, short shins; long shins, short femurs), the net product will be a high hip position that will benefit from being a bit lower down. In the case of long femurs, the hip position is made worse because the longer femur length will place the hip joint (the axis) farther away from the barbell. The likely outcome—especially if the torso is of average length or shorter—is a shoulder position that is behind the barbell in space rather than directly above it. Most of the time, the compensation for this situation comes in the form of added dorsiflexion to position the bar under the shoulders. Longer shins and shorter femurs may make for a better shoulder position relative to the bar, but the severe hip flexion can result in a desperate need for long arms to make the lift a success. If they aren't part of the lifter's anatomy, problems can ensue in the form of—you guessed it—spinal curvature.

Round-Back Deadlift

We're about to completely contradict what we wrote earlier about spinal posture for the deadlift in this section. Bear with us.

Traditional wisdom dictates that the spine remain extended or neutral when deadlifting. Very little research has been conducted about the effects of lifting with a more rounded spine. However, some of the strongest athletes in the world lift with a flexed spine. In general, a maximal lift will pull the athlete's spine into some degree of flexion. Many deadlift athletes intentionally choose a round-back posture and are able to lift extremely heavy loads in this manner without issue.

McGill, McDermott, and Fenwick (2009) note that in a comparison of strongman events (yoke, Atlas stone, farmer carry, keg carry, tire flip, and log press), the Atlas stone yielded the least compressive forces on the lumbar spine despite the flexed spinal position required by the lift. The general reasoning is twofold:

1. The lift required "low spine power," in the words of the study authors. In other words, the spine did not move much in the initial stone lift—the only real change was at the top of the lift, once the stone was ready to be placed.

2. The stone remained extremely close to the torso during the lift, thus reducing risk of injury.

In the deadlift, a rounded back changes the leverages of the body so that the bar can travel in the straightest vertical line possible. In this manner, the bar is as close to the body as it can be. Although it isn't on top of the torso the way an Atlas stone might be, keeping the bar close to the body reduces risk of injury to the lumbar spine.

Mawston and colleagues (2021) performed a small study (to our knowledge the only one of its kind) on flexing the spine when lifting. The authors found that a flexed spine increased strength and efficiency in a maximal lift. While this study did not examine risk of injury using a round-back stance, it implies that using this position may be an advantage for pain-free athletes.

All this considered, a round-back deadlift should likely be employed by athletes who already have high levels of torso strength and who are adept at deadlifting. Traditional advice of keeping the spine slightly lordotic or neutral when training the deadlift is likely wise while learning the lift and gaining strength.

That said, the round-back deadlift may be of particular interest to athletes with long torsos or long legs, who may have more trouble creating a position in which they can pull the barbell in a fully vertical line. This type of posture might also help these athletes lift more weight than they might otherwise be able to manage.

Best Variation: Medium Sumo Barbell Deadlift

The simple modification of freeing the legs from obstruction by the arms can be a liberating change that the body needs—regardless of which of the three body types the lifter possesses. For big lifters, this modification does two things: First, it can provide more clearance for the trunk space to fit between the legs (no blockage from the abdominal region when hinging over), and second, it can better align the feet and legs with the acetabula so the lifter isn't forcing a stance narrower than their natural sweet spot.

For lifters with long shins, consider the difference in back angles between the medium sumo deadlift setup (figure 5.7a and b) and a conventional deadlift setup (figure 5.7c and d). The torso is allowed to stay significantly more

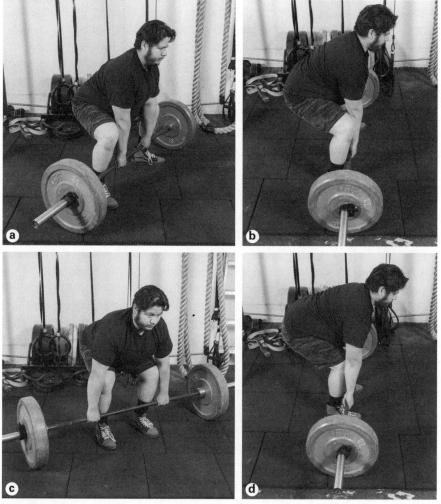

FIGURE 5.7   Sumo squat deadlift: start position, front view (a) and side view (b); conventional deadlift: start position, front view (c), and side view (d).

upright when pulling medium sumo because of the added space afforded to the hips to drop down. It creates more ease in finding the right position over the bar and sinking down slightly deeper than normal (which can be of benefit if the lifter's arms aren't all that long). Moreover, for lifters with long femurs, the added space can ensure a vertical shin position while still accommodating the requirement of the scapulae to be above the barbell in space.

Something of note when switching to what's essentially a squat stance with a barbell deadlift is the issue of knurling and chafing. A typical Olympic barbell (and many other kinds of 45-pound [20 kg] barbells) will have knurling (rough textured grips) on most of the barbell, less the middle portion. Some barbells will have a strip of center knurling also, with smooth areas to the left and right of that center knurling. With the medium sumo stance, the hands will more than likely be positioned on a part of the bar that is without knurling, whereas the shins, which when conventionally oriented are against a smooth surface, will now be placed against knurled areas of the bar. Unfortunately, this can lead to a poorer quality hand grip as well as abrasions and scrapes along the shins as the reps progress.

Our advice would be to deadlift with pants, high socks, or shin sleeves if preparing to deadlift with this variation to avoid bruising or bleeding, and to select a bar with the most knurling closest to the middle of the bar so at least part of the hands can benefit from the added grip. Using chalk can be helpful to an extent, but as reps begin to get heavier, a lifter can consider using a mixed grip if necessary.

Do not get this stance confused with a full, wide sumo stance. The reason the full sumo stance is not listed as a recommended alternative in this book is because it's typically used only for shortening the bar's path and for its training benefits to muscles. The wide sumo stance requires that the feet be kept extremely far apart, in some cases almost as wide as the plates on either end of the barbell. Although this may work for some lifters in the pursuit of lifting more weight, it's not friendly to the hip region because of the severe external femoral rotation under load. In keeping with the ideas we've presented, it's ideal for the femurs to line up with the acetabula when performing a loaded pattern. For most people, it's unlikely this wide stance accomplishes that objective. For proof, look to the field. Many times, the first area of weakness or breach that a sumo deadlifter experiences comes in the form of the knees caving in, disrupting the alignment between ankle and hip. There's a definite reason for this, and it's not just tight adductors.

For these reasons, we recommend the medium sumo position. It's safer and a more realistic way to pull as a modification of the conventional setup.

Kettlebell Deadlift

What this movement variation lacks in the amount of absolute weight one can lift it makes up for in the number of customizations big lifters, or lifters with different lower limb proportions, can benefit from (figure 5.8*a-b*). A lifter will be hard pressed to find a kettlebell that weighs much more than 110 pounds (50 kg) in their gym—but even using one (or a pair) of these weights allows a lifter to find an uninhibited medium sumo leg position while still holding on with a narrow grip (which can be turned to neutral for even more comfort). Most kettlebells have great grips on the handles (solving the knurling issue), and the weights can be positioned farther between the feet or farther away from the body as needed to accommodate for longer femurs.

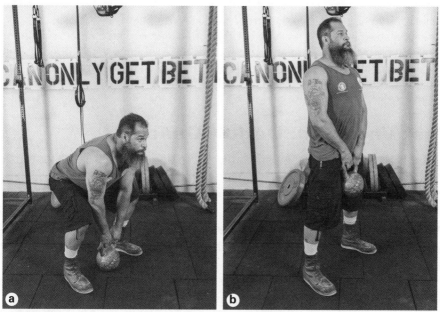

FIGURE 5.8   Single kettlebell deadlift: start position *(a)*, and finish *(b)*.

Deadlifting: Short, With Small Hands

Having a compact frame and a short overall body usually translates itself to plenty of strength thanks to the shorter distance the bar must travel in a given movement. This may be true, but for a lifter looking for increased time under tension to better work target muscles, this truth can be of equal frustration. The good news is that, because of the shorter pulling space, reaching down for a barbell at standard elevation is going to be less of an ask for a lifter's mobility and flexibility—in other words, it's unlikely to be as difficult a task to get into the proper starting position when you're a shorter lifter.

Barbell Thickness and Deadlifts

It's not uncommon to associate a smaller overall body with smaller hands and feet. One often comes with the other. For that reason, it's useful to go over one important side note before we continue.

A standard men's Olympic barbell has a thickness of 1.1 inches (28 mm) in diameter. For some smaller lifters with smaller hands, that can feel like the equivalent of a larger, taller lifter holding on to an axle bar or using fat grips. And it's not conducive to a strong pull performance. It can be downright frustrating to know the muscles of your body aren't near fatigue but the muscles of the hands and forearms just can't get in the game.

By contrast, a women's Olympic bar has a diameter of 0.98 inches (25 mm). This may not sound like a significant difference by the numbers, but it's one that a lifter will instantly feel with bar in hand. Whether male or female, making the switch to a women's Olympic bar for deadlifts can be a smart choice for training purposes and adding much-needed lifting volume while reducing grip fatigue. Although the women's bar is 12 pounds (5 kg) lighter and about half a foot shorter, accounting for this when calculating load is a very simple task.

Best Variation: Deficit Deadlift

Pulling the barbell from a raised platform creates added time under tension, which a shorter lifter can benefit from when available range of motion isn't on their side. A platform anywhere from 2 inches (5 cm) high to 8 inches (20 cm) high makes for a deeper starting position, while still relying on the lifter's flexibility and mobility to achieve a properly extended spine in the set position. (Of note: If a lifter cannot achieve this position, then it's not worth using the deficit deadlift until said position can be achieved.) The lifter stands on the platform, with the loaded barbell situated on the floor, so the feet will be closer to the bar, vertically speaking (figure 5.9a). The added inches of pulling space may not seem like much on a single rep, but it definitely adds up as volume is increased over the course of a workout session.

As you can see, the main requirement of a deficit deadlift in terms of choosing an appropriate surface is making sure said surface is stable and unmoving (figure 5.9b). Second—and obviously—the platform should not be so wide that the plates of the loaded bar are resting on it at the bottom position, because this would defeat the purpose. Commonly, lifters will stand on low step platforms or large weight plates.

As a bonus, deficit deadlifts and their added time under tension mean more time spent holding onto the bar, which can have a positive impact on the training effect received by the forearm flexors and hand musculature to aid grip strength. Moreover, small-handed lifters need more grip training in order to keep the bar tightly in grasp (especially with a double overhand grip). In this case, using the touch-and-go method mentioned earlier allows

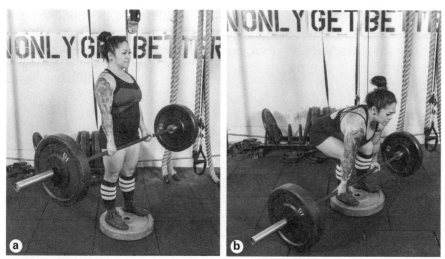

FIGURE 5.9   Deficit deadlift: start position *(a)*, and finish *(b)*.

the lifter to maintain tension throughout the entire set and not have a break in grip strength. Some may see this as a disadvantage and a recipe for early fatigue, but it's important to consider it from the opposite perspective—that of training a weak link.

If You Have No Platform

For some, the platforms they have to pull from can be either too high or not the right surface to stand on (e.g., uneven). In this case, smaller weight plates can come in handy. For example, a 25- or 35-pound (12 or 16 kg) iron plate is typically smaller in diameter than a 45-pound (20 kg) plate (figure 5.10). Loading two 25-pound plates on a bar instead of one 45-pound plate equals greater load, but the bar will be lower to the ground. If you're stuck with nothing to elevate your feet on, just resort to lowering the bar instead.

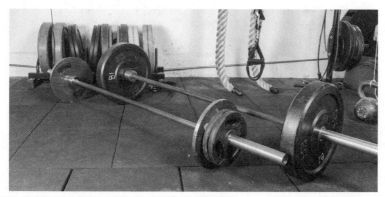

FIGURE 5.10   Different weight barbells change the distance of reach for the lifter.

Since shorter deadlifters don't have the problems of time under tension and distance traveled that taller or longer-legged deadlifters might, it's less likely they'll be affected by high volume in the deadlift pattern itself. For that reason, aggressive volume measures can be taken, as long as ample rest intervals are respected.

Snatch Grip Deadlift

Using a wide grip to perform deadlifts can be another alternative to create more pulling range of motion. A typical snatch grip would have the bar sitting in the fold of the hip when the arms are fully extended while the body is in a standing position, but it doesn't have to be that severe. Even widening the hand position by 6 to 8 inches (15-20 cm) on either side creates a noteworthy change in pulling space and required body geometry (figure 5.11a). With a wider grip, a lifter is forced into a double overhand position because there's no way to use a mixed grip with the arms wide. Furthermore, it adds greater involvement of another muscle group into the mix: the latissimus dorsi (lats).

Keep in mind that the lats are an internal rotator of the upper arm. Carrying load in a wide overhand grip relies on their engagement through the pattern, as the shoulder extends and the bar is raised off the ground while the body straightens. The lats' involvement in the deadlift is important, regardless of the version of the deadlift in question. The lifter's ability to create adequate tension on the bar via the lats' engagement will be a difference maker in keeping the bar close to the body and ensuring an upright bar path. In addition, since the hands are out wide in a snatch grip position, the natural tendency will be to squeeze the hands inward (toward each other) to create tension and a strong grip. In addition to internal rotation, the lats' role is also adduction of the upper

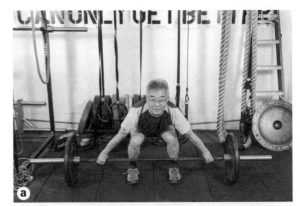

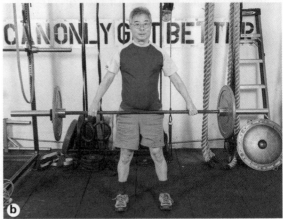

FIGURE 5.11   Snatch grip deadlift: start position *(a)*, and finish *(b)*.

arm, meaning even more activity from this wide position compared with a typical conventional deadlift (figure 5.11b).

As a bonus, if you don't have anything but bumper plates in your gym setup (or are stuck with only 45 pound [20 kg] iron plates), widening the grip can replicate the need for greater range of motion when pulling. Even when the difference is a few vital inches, it could mean everything when it comes to a workout containing sets and reps.

Deadlift Training Volume

Research indicates that changing between conventional deadlifts, trap bar deadlifts, and even hip thrusts creates no noteworthy difference in lumbar region activity and erector spinae involvement (Andersen et al. 2018)—but these findings are contingent on the body types of the individuals who underwent testing. People who can achieve a similar torso angle using a barbell as they would using a trap bar will certainly see similar amounts of lumbar region demand from lift to lift. For lifters who are faced with a more horizontal torso position in their conventional deadlift setup, it's crucial to consider the amount of volume and forces they endure in the lumbar region compared with another lifter. Five sets of 10 reps while lifting a body-weight equivalent deadlift will be a very different experience for the lumbar region of two lifters if lifter A has a back angle of 40 degrees relative to the floor and lifter B has a back angle of 85 degrees relative to the floor.

Each lifter, because of their anthropometry, would be setting up for and performing the deadlift correctly for their body type, but that doesn't mean the demands of the movement would be the same for these lifters. Good technique may be more universally linear compared with training effect delivered. The lifter with the 85-degree back angle would be deeper hinged to maintain a fairly vertical shin, likely meaning a taller overall height, shorter arms, longer legs or femurs, or a shorter torso (or a combination of these). It's in proper order to consider these demands and adjust volume and lift intensity accordingly.

The first area to be addressed is prescribed rest between sets. Especially during heavier work sets, adding 15 to 20 percent longer rest intervals can be helpful to reduce injury risk due to under-recovery between sets, specifically for the lumbar region. Second, changing lifting volume to suit these particulars could involve fewer sets at top loads while focusing more on adding volume to ramping sets.

When it comes to volume, people tend to think in very strict terms: More volume equals more sets and total reps of an exercise. Although that's not wrong, there's more to it than that.

In the scenario of a deadlift workout where a lifter is planning to do five sets of 8 reps at a working weight of 300 pounds (135 kg), said lifter would be smart to ramp their way up to the 300-pound mark rather than put it all on the bar for the first set. A ramp-up might look something like this:

95 lb (45 kg) × 5 reps
135 lb (60 kg) × 3 reps
185 lb (85 kg) × 2 reps
205 lb (95 kg) × 2 reps
225 lb (100 kg) × 2 reps
250 lb (115 kg) × 2 reps
275 lb (125 kg) × 2 reps
300 lb (135 kg) × 8 × 5 sets

If you do the math, the cumulative weight lifted comes out to 15,160 pounds (6,845 kg) spread across 58 reps. But the chances of running out of steam or hitting the endurance wall is pretty high—let alone what five sets of 8 reps at 300 pounds after all that ramping might risk for the lower back, based on the demographic in question. Especially for high-frequency training, adding volume to all ramping sets while performing only one or two max sets may sound like a much less demanding endeavor, but using the same weights, it would look like this:

95 lb (45 kg) × 8 reps
135 lb (60 kg) × 8 reps
185 lb (85 kg) × 8 reps
205 lb (95 kg) × 8 reps
225 lb (100 kg) × 8 reps
250 lb (115 kg) × 8 reps
275 lb (125 kg) × 8 reps
300 lb (135 kg) × 8 × 2 sets

Here, the total is 15,760 pounds (7,160 kg) spread across 72 reps. In this example, the lifter will have performed 8 reps for every ramping set but will also be able to remain more technically sound because the ramping sets aren't pushing the threshold of the lifter's 8-rep max. This trick allows the lifter to do more work submaximally, without getting crushed under heavy weights that place the lower back at higher risk. Especially for the purposes of muscular development, this method is a smart one to employ.

Key Drills for Better Deadlifts

Since the hip region and spine are key players in successful deadlifts, it makes sense that the most mobilization patterns will be centered around these regions to promote the best possible performance. Each of these drills is smart to incorporate into warm-ups or between sets for best results, regardless of the body type of the lifter.

Hip Rockbacks

Deep hip flexion requires good hip mobility while maintaining a neutral spine. This drill addresses this demand and was mentioned in chapter 2 (see page 22).

Dowel Hinge Pattern

The lifter holds a dowel vertically behind the back, aiming for the head, upper back, and glutes to be in contact with it. The top hand should hold the dowel (palm in) behind the neck. The bottom hand should hold the dowel (palm out) behind the lower back. Maintaining all three points of contact, the lifter folds at the hip joint, pushing the glutes backward and keeping the spine extended. The moment one of the points of contact can't be maintained, they stop the rep, readjust, and perform the next rep, moving slowly through all phases.

Glute Bridge

Lying flat on the back, the lifter bends the knees to 90-degree angles while the heels remain flat on the floor. After removing any space from under the low back (it should be flush with the ground), the lifter squeezes the glutes while engaging the abs. Next, they raise the hips to full extension, creating a straight line from shoulder to knee. They hold for one second, then lower slowly. Repeat for sets of 12 to 15 reps.

Ideal Supplementary Lifts to Aid the Deadlift

Supplementary lifts may not mimic the exact pattern of the deadlift itself, but they involve the same muscle groups and exploit body positions that prove useful for strengthening the deadlift. For lifters who want to improve their deadlift performance and strength, these movements should be included somewhere in programming. This goes for all body types, because the contraindications that deadlifts may present for certain body types are drastically reduced or eliminated thanks to force angles, loading quantities, or implements used.

- Reverse hyperextension
- Horizontal back extension
- Barbell hip thrust
- Dumbbell single-leg deadlift
- Cable pull-through

The deadlift is indeed one of the most useful and popular patterns among the big lifts. The size of this chapter alone and the options that exist within it show just how individualized the approach needs to be when programming the deadlift. Remember: This movement most directly involves the lumbar spine, and it's the single lift that carries the highest potential for the most weight to be moved. With that said, it's important to play it safe and err on the side of caution, while implementing the right modifications to suit your clients' body types.

Chapter 6

The Squat Pattern

Although similar in overall nature, the difference between a deadlift pattern and a squat pattern is that the latter is a knee-dominant movement. That simply means a greater amount of knee flexion (or knee bending) is required to perform squat variations compared with deadlift variations. As such, the two exercises have different training effects, and despite a few similarities, there is little crossover effect between squats and deadlifts in their conventional form (Hales, Johnson, and Johnson 2009). There are countless squat variations because of how universal—and important—a movement it is. That makes it even more useful to review what squat versions fit best for the demographic in question based on body type. But first, let's look at the squat-friendly anthropometry.

The Perfect Barbell Squat Body Type

As mentioned in chapter 3 on fundamental movement patterns, for the purposes of clarity and consistency, we refer to the barbell back squat as the conventional, standard version of the squat. We chose this simply because it's the most commonly used squat variation and typically one of the most accessible barbell variations for people who lift. Anatomy of the hips plays a large role in just how deep a person can squat, but proportions can be important to consider for the same purposes. Whereas the deadlift pattern places the focus on how far the bar travels away from the floor, to measure how much work (remember, work equals force times distance) is performed, we believe it's smarter to look at how far the hip joint descends to get a similar idea when considering the squat. For that reason, a greater distance traveled by the hip joint (a longer descent and ascent to achieve a deep depth) will mean more work for the lifter. In the name of efficiency and strength, adding work per rep may not be ideal. Hence, this lends to the idea that a shorter pair of legs is a blessing where squatting is concerned, because the distance between point A and point B for the hips to travel will be limited.

Notice we specified only shorter legs. The reason is that we must consider the geometrical angles assumed by the upper body in order to promote minimal stress forces on the lumbar spine. If a lifter is short overall, with proportionate balances between the lower and upper body, the torso needs to be angled to a certain degree of hip flexion in order to keep the bar positioned over the middle of the foot in space. For most people of congruent proportions, this results in the shin angle matching or closely comparing to the torso angle at the bottom position of the squat. With that said, a longer torso means a more upright torso angle at the bottom of the squat in order to achieve the same balance. Assuming the barbell is in the same position on the back, the hip joint is able to maintain a slightly larger angle, meaning lesser stress forces for the lumbar region to endure. In the field, we find this to hold true when considering Olympic lifters at the elite levels and their pervasive body types. Pound for pound, these are undoubtedly the strongest full-range squatters in the world, and interestingly, the body types don't show much variation, regardless of the weight class of the lifter.

Since the arms and hands don't move while performing a squat, they're less important in defining the ideal squatting body type. A body that has a longer torso, shorter legs, and adequate requisite mobility—including an ideal hip anatomy to support proper hip range of motion (a more open acetabular space that may be more front facing than side facing)—will be conducive to strong, deep, injury- and pain-free squats; this is a great starting point to build from. For lifters with other body types, they may be in for a few challenges to make the movement work well for them.

Squatting: Short Torso and Long Legs; Long Femurs; Tall

The main issue that lifters in these three body categories have is being able to achieve a full range of motion and a deeper depth. Lifters in the tall category may not have any glaring disproportion that's clearly visible, but the sheer distance they need to travel can demand a lot of their mobility and energy, which can make the back squat pattern a challenge. Poor mobility in a squat usually results in at least one of the following compensations:

1. The hips don't sink enough, and as a result, the torso pitches forward to make up for lost space. This results in greater load bearing for the lower back.

2. The heels rise off the ground or begin to slide out of position compared with their starting point. This is another compensation that happens when proper stability cannot be established through bottom end ranges.

3. The lumbar spine goes through noteworthy flexion due to posterior pelvic tilting. This happens when a lifter who is not mobile or flexible enough "reaches" for a range of motion that is unattainable. This severe butt wink can be dangerous and injurious if not monitored.

Lifters in these demographics who are plagued by one or more of these issues typically need a less severe torso angle and improved mobility at the ankle and hip joints to ameliorate the situation. Looking for the congruency between torso and shin angle as mentioned earlier is a good place to start and may require variations that better fit the lifter and their body.

Best Variation: Barbell Front Squat

It's truly amazing just how many issues can be addressed by simply switching from a back squat to a front squat. The first thing it does is force the lifter to consider the physics. Since the squat is a vertical push pattern (a lifter pushes the bar away from the floor to complete the squat), the ideal bar position is over the middle of the foot (we've been over this, as you know). In motion, the bar should travel in as straight a line as possible to maximize movement efficiency and minimize disturbances to its path. Knowing this, consider the starting position of a back squat. Most would be quick to conclude that standing with the bar positioned on the back equals an upright, completely vertical starting position, with the hips open to a 180-degree angle—and they would be wrong.

For the bar to be balanced on the back at the start of a back squat, the hips need to start flexed with the torso angled slightly forward by a few inches. This not only keeps the bar from rolling off the back but also places the bar in the right place in space. This creates a greater propensity to push the hips back to initiate the squat, which can counter the necessary mechanics for people of the body type demographics being spoken of. For them, the reliance on knee bend may be greater than for shorter-legged lifters, because the rate of angular change required at the knee joint in order for its flexion to keep up with hip flexion will be faster compared with a lifter with shorter legs. If this didn't happen, the excessive hip flexion would result in a severely angled torso and the issue discussed in point 1, listed earlier.

Placing the loaded barbell on the front of the body instead of the back of the body allows a lifter to truly open up the hips for a true tall starting position. Remember: The bar's placement over the midfoot means the upper body will be able to remain behind the bar at the top, rather than in front of it. Since the weight is acting as more of a counterbalance in this setup, it allows the lifter to better sit against the weight and to initiate the squat from more of a simultaneous knee and hip flexion (knee flexion may even start an instant before hip flexion). All of this will promote a deeper depth, when all things are equal. It will also reduce lumbar region stress, compared with a back squat (Fuglsang, Telling, and Sørensen 2017). Plus, the front squat creates certain lifting terms: If you pitch forward too far, the bar is coming down. That creates a greater demand for the torso to remain vertical, forcing the lumbar spine to endure less shear.

To perform a successful full-range front squat, a lifter will be best off when having a good degree of dorsiflexion, wrist and shoulder mobility, and thoracic spine extension. For all of these reasons, a front squat proves itself to be a generally more athletically demanding variation of the two barbell squats—and one that emphasizes the proper function of most load-bearing joints.

Types of Grips for Front Squats

Front squats can be performed by holding the barbell in either a clean grip (figure 6.1*a*) or a bodybuilding-style cross-armed grip, also known as the California style (figure 6.1*b*).

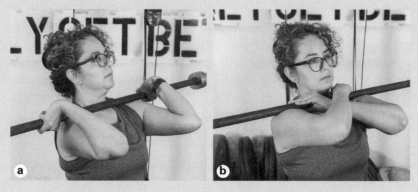

Figure 6.1   Barbell grips: clean *(a)*, and California *(b)*.

The clean grip is the one we recommend, for a reason similar to why we recommend a double overhand deadlifting grip. In the case of the front squat, using a clean grip ensures the shoulders and elbows stay at the same level, potentiating more balance throughout the body and decreasing the chance of cascading imbalances or dominance issues while performing the movement under load. Furthermore, the California-style grip can be a bit finicky; the bar is more likely to slide away from the neck area and down the deltoid toward the upper arm as the elbows drop and the lifter performs repetitions. Having adequate thoracic extension while using a clean grip (with the fingers holding the bar and the thumb free) can keep the bar from sliding forward and create a better shelf for it to rest on. The goal should be to maintain tension on the barbell by pulling upward with the elbows and hands the entire time.

If a lifter doesn't have adequate mobility to keep the elbows high using the clean grip, there are drills that can help. A thoracic extension is performed by lying on top of a foam roller placed widthwise under the thoracic spine (figure 6.2). Without raising the hips, the goal is to extend the spine around the roller while arching the midback (not the lower back).

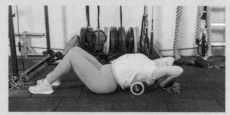

Figure 6.2   Foam roller extensions.

Performing this for sets of 6 to 12 reps before starting workouts and between sets can help train the spine to assume the correct posture when in action.

Front Squatting for Lifters With Lots of Muscle Mass (Big All Over)

Assuming a clean grip or even a California grip can often be problematic for big lifters who are looking to front squat, the usual reason being a lack of space to hold onto the bar because of too much overall mass. Most com-

monly, we've seen lifters with very large arms (who might be on the shorter side also) unable to assume a clean grip simply because their biceps block their hands from getting there when the bar is on the torso. For that reason, it may be unrealistic to force a standard front squat grip on said lifter. A simple hack, however, is to use straps to hold the barbell up, which lets the lifter comfortably keep the weight in the correct rack position without needing to have the hands directly connected to the bar, giving the clearance needed to keep the elbows up (figure 6.3).

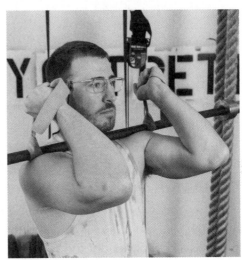

FIGURE 6.3 Front squat rack position using straps.

Heels-Elevated Dumbbell Squat

For lifters in the categories of tall, long legs, and long femurs, a full range of motion squat will be heavily contingent on the lifter's ability to dorsiflex. The longer a lifter's legs are relative to the rest of the body, the more dorsiflexion that lifter will need for the hips to drop below knee level with the spine remaining relatively vertical. Since the front squat's loading is on the anterior side of the body, the knees will cross forward over the toes more to accomplish the lift. If the lifter's ankle mobility is lacking, however, more of the same problems will present themselves in the form of pitching forward at the torso and the elbows dropping or heels lifting.

A lack of dorsiflexion capability can be mitigated by elevating the heels—in this case, much higher than can be accomplished by a typical Olympic lifting shoe or standing on thin weight plates. Using a slant board or wedge to put the full foot on a grade makes for a much more severe heel elevation, placing the foot in a very plantar-flexed position (figure 6.4a). Since the rest of the body remains vertical, squatting from this starting position means there's much more available room for dorsiflexion because the joint angle at the ankle starts in a deficit (or a much larger angle than when on flat ground). All of this means the knees will be allowed to travel forward without the heel of the foot rising away from its surface, and the spine will be able to remain upright (figure 6.4b).

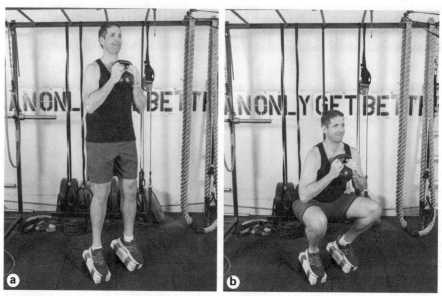

FIGURE 6.4   Squat on slant board: start position *(a)*, and finish *(b)*.

Of note, squatting like this will certainly bias the quadriceps as target muscles, since the degree of knee flexion compared with the degree of hip flexion will be in favor of the knees, and hence the knee extensors (quadriceps) will have plenty of activity. Later in this chapter, we discuss ways to get more contribution from the posterior chain when squatting with long femurs.

To add dumbbells to the heels-elevated squat, the lifter would hold dumbbells by the sides, like two suitcases (figure 6.5*a*). This doubles as a way to squat when a lifter might not be mobile or flexible enough in the upper body

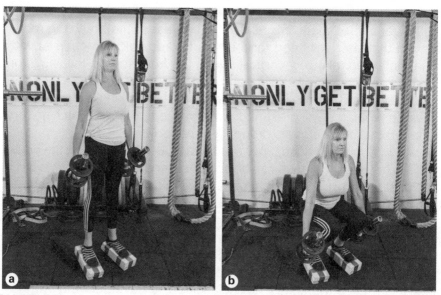

FIGURE 6.5   Heels-elevated dumbbell squat: start position *(a)*, and finish *(b)*.

for a front rack position. Aiming to keep the body upright while descending and simultaneously looking for the dumbbells to land right beside the ankles on each descent will ensure a good-quality heels-elevated dumbbell squat (figure 6.5b). Using a slant board or wedge will probably force the feet to be narrower than the lifter's normal squat stance, but this will be within the realms of possibility since the elevated heels will create much better clearance for the narrow-stance squat to be achieved with no compensations.

Squatting: Long Shins; Short

Having longer shins when squatting will mean less reliance on dorsiflexion and a likely limit to just how much range of motion can be attained when squatting deep. Similarly, a lifter with a short overall height may be looking for more time under tension when squatting in order to get the most out of the muscles despite a small overall range of motion. Squatting to a box or to partial ranges will still provide benefits for lifters, but it may not optimize and make best use of the particulars of the anthropometrics of lifters in these categories.

Especially for these body types, it's even more important to determine just what squat stance will promote the best overall range of motion. Trial and error when squatting, along with the hip rockback drill on page 22, will help you do this. Once that's been established, adding time spent dealing with the load should be a priority.

Best Variation: Slow, Eccentric Paused Back Squat

There's not much esoteric science to explain this exercise and its benefits to a lifter: Adding seconds to the eccentric component of a squat increases the amount of time spent bearing the load. Including a two- or three- second pause eliminates any transfers of forces and momentum to be used during the lift. This makes the lift more honest but also forces a lifter to dial in on focus and maintain tension through the entire body.

Of note, it's very easy to relax at the bottom of a paused squat and let the body sit in the fully flexed position without any concerted contraction. It's worth remembering that muscles connect to joints via tendons. If the muscles aren't as active as possible—especially through end ranges—it can lead to joint laxity and the susceptibility to injury. Since joints often get injured while they're changing positions, it's up to the muscles of the body to bolster them through a controlled pattern like an exercise in the weight room. Deliberately activating more muscles that surround a joint (in order to better support that joint) is the textbook definition of the law of irradiation, which states that recruitment of neighboring muscles to a working muscle can amplify the strength and stability of the movement in question.

Isometric Squat

Similar to the isometric deadlift in chapter 5 (p. 73), using isometrics isn't just a way to increase time under tension. It also reduces injury risk while strengthening parts of a force curve that most lifters would simply pass through. In the case of shorter lifters, or lifters with depth limitations due to their lower limb anthropometry, this is a great choice to supplement their programming. This isn't a simple act of body-weight squatting to full depth and pausing there for a period of time, however; contracting maximally is lacking from this example. Instead, set up a safety bar at a lifter's bottom range (or set up a supramaximally loaded barbell on pins at that bottom range). The lifter sets up under the bar in a deep squat position and applies maximal tension—once again assuming the bar cannot be moved—to drive up against the bar in an attempt to "stand up with the weight," aiming for sets of 15- to 30-second holds.

Using this method for various squatting knee joint angles can be a useful way to stimulate the nervous system to potentiate strength improvement while fatiguing the muscles in an ideal fashion to potentiate hypertrophy. We recommend this isometric training method in conjunction with typical isotonic exercise. We do not believe that strength or development gains come strictly from isometric training; it should supplement the workout program. In the case of lifters who have these particular hindrances to their squat pattern, it is fine for it to take up a slightly larger portion of training, although traditional training methods should still have their place.

Squatting: Big All Over

A big lifter with a heavy scale weight usually has mobility limitations. For that reason, it may be a hassle to set up for typical back squats and front squats or to find the right technique. This immobility usually presents itself in a couple of ways:

1. Poor shoulder mobility prevents a proper rack position for front squats or causes torquing of the elbows when reaching back for back squats.
2. Poor hip mobility due to trunk volume leads to a naturally wider stance to assume better clearance (this way the abdominal region doesn't block the legs from achieving deeper knee flexion).

Regardless of a lifter's height, these restrictions tend to remain in place and can be frustrating for a lifter who may otherwise have a good squat and good strength. To start, it's imperative that lifters who fit this category get the most out of their own levels of mobility, notwithstanding their size. The squat mobility drill can help prepare all lifters for a squatting workout, but we believe it is even more useful for lifters in this category. To perform this drill, a lifter descends to a deep squat with the foot width comfortable for them. They can disregard their spine position (it doesn't have to be neutral; for the purposes of the drill, rounding is acceptable). Once at the bottom squatting position, driving the elbows in between the knees and gently pushing them outward is the next step. While in this position it's ideal to attempt to sit taller by raising the rib cage and engaging the postural muscles of the middle and upper back. Third, the lifter plants both hands on the ground just inside the feet and raises one hand toward the ceiling, making sure to rotate the upper body toward that side. The arm with the hand still planted on the floor will block the knee on that side from caving inward. The lifter then switches arms and repeats before standing. Performing as many reps as needed can help a lifter reach their potential before any squat exercises. With this in mind, it's time to consider the squat variation we feel is the most fitting for big lifters.

Best Variation: Safety Bar Squat

Anecdotally, we've found that using a safety bar tends to make a lifter gravitate toward a wider foot position, which is consistent for bigger lifters. More importantly, however, the safety bar differs from a barbell in the way it's secured. It's a back-loaded exercise (the bar still rests on the traps), but its yoke design features handles that are held in front of the body, in a much lower position compared with a back or front squat. This modification is a real shoulder and elbow saver for lifters who experience frustration with barbell work, and it can often result in a deeper squatting depth because less of that depth is contingent on keeping the bar in the right place on the upper back. In the case of a front squat, for example, a lifter might have the lower body mobility to squat deep, but the thoracic spine or shoulder mobility may not be at the same level, causing the elbows to drop prematurely, the bar to move forward (with the torso following suit) during the squat itself, and an insufficient depth as a result of all this while the lifter struggles to maintain efficiency.

In the case of a back squat, many big lifters resort to a low bar position (where the bar is placed lower on the scapulae rather than the meatier part of the upper traps). This difference of a few inches can drastically affect the geometry in a back squat. Mentioned earlier in the chapter, the hips aren't completely extended in the start and finish position of a back squat. The bar must remain over the midfoot, meaning the torso needs to lean forward to accommodate this. When the bar is lower down the back, the torso needs to lean forward to a corresponding degree. This means less hip extension, greater trunk lean during the squat, and a shallower potential for depth achieved in the lift.

To ameliorate this, the safety bar allows for a high bar position, without the restraints just listed. Since the elbows can be comfortably positioned down by the lifter's sides (figure 6.6), a lifter can place more focus on the lower body's mobility and achieve a better depth with a more upright torso. With that said, a lifter would do well to remember that tension still applies to the safety bar, even though the hands are on handles and not on the bar itself. Packing the shoulders down to engage the upper back is a smart thing to do, and determining the optimal position for the elbows and handles is also important. Some of this depends on a lifter's comfort level, but some also depends on arm length. Big lifters with longer arms may prefer a position where the safety handles are angled slightly away from the body (upward) rather than pointing straight down. This hand position will still slightly raise the elbows and keep them from making contact with the thighs or knees on the descent (figure 6.7), which would otherwise hinder range of motion. Depending on the length of the safety handles (these can vary from bar to bar), this can be a pivotal adjustment. Similarly, allowing the elbows to bow outward slightly can do the same to avoid intersection with the arms and legs. This depends on

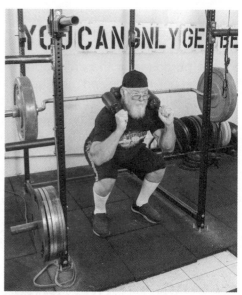

FIGURE 6.6 Midphase of safety bar squat.

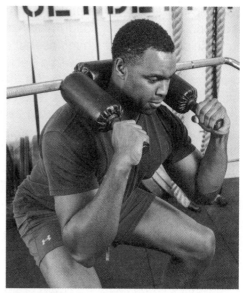

FIGURE 6.7 Safety bar squat with higher elbow position.

both the foot width assumed by the lifter and the distance between handles on the safety bar, because both can vary.

It's worth noting that safety bars vary in weight but are usually all heavier than a standard 45-pound (20 kg) Olympic bar. The typical lower end in weight that we've seen for safety bars has been 65 pounds (30 kg).

Frankenstein Squat

The subsection dedicated to front squatting for big lifters suggested using straps as one trick for front-loaded squats, and the Frankenstein squat is another that won't sacrifice loading. The Frankenstein squat forces the body to remain upright while performing a hands-free variation of the exercise. It sounds like something that would severely limit the amount a lifter can move, but in truth, it simply takes some getting used to. To do this variation, a lifter sets up under the bar by placing it on the front of the body behind the deltoids. The bar will be up near the neck, ideally nested in the natural notch between the neck and shoulder (figure 6.8a). Once the load is unracked, the lifter will carefully remove the hands from the bar and place the arms straight out in front, angled slightly upward. It is imperative that nothing compromise this position; the elbows should not bend, and the hands should not drop downward for the entire set (figure 6.8b). Keeping the hands neutral (palms facing each other) and the fists clenched can help with this tension.

This hand and arm position acts as a counterbalance, since some of the lifter's body weight is now positioned farther away from the body than normal. All of this can accentuate a taller and more upright squatting position, which is conducive to greater range of motion. Adding a pause at the bottom of each rep can help the lifter maintain control over the weight and ensure a consistent bar path. It's recommended to keep reps low; five reps per set is plenty here. This can be a reasonable option for lifters who don't have access to a safety bar.

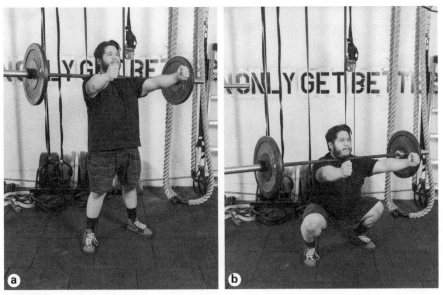

FIGURE 6.8   Frankenstein squat: start position (a), and finish (b).

Hip Belt Squat

Hip belt squatting stations are less common to come by; this piece of equipment is mostly purchased by performance-oriented gyms, often in the powerlifting or bodybuilding community. Using a hip belt takes the hands and arms out of the picture completely, while sparing the spine of excessive stress forces thanks to the lack of axial loading (Joseph et al. 2020). In truth, it's an excellent choice for bigger lifters who lack mobility for traditional squatting methods.

When using an actual hip belt squat machine, the load the lifter can apply can rival a heavy barbell or safety bar squat, since there are usually full-sized plate-loading columns on either side or a full pin stack to select from, depending on the make and model of the machine.

Hip belt squat machines have a rail that faces the lifter, allowing for mild hand guidance through the movement to keep the lifter focused on the mechanics of the lift and the lower body bias this squat variation can offer (figure 6.9a). Because of the lower body isolation, this variation is better suited for higher reps than for lower reps, possibly even as a secondary movement to one of the main lifts. Again, a lifter won't achieve full hip extension using this method, since the harness for the load goes around the lower back region. That can be beneficial if the lifter's goal is to save the muscles of the lumbar region like the erector spinae and quadratus lumborum from being involved in spinal extension. The torso angle achieved will still place plenty of mechanical tension on the hamstrings and glutes, however, especially in the bottom positions of the exercise (figure 6.9b).

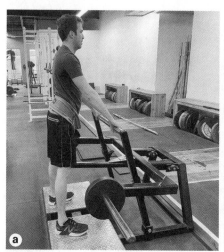 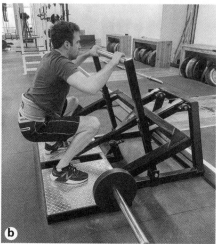

FIGURE 6.9 Hip belt squat: start position *(a)*, and finish *(b)*.

Hip Belt Squat Alternative: Weight Belt Squat

As mentioned, the hip belt squat machine is a more difficult find in the gym world, and if you don't have access to one, there are makeshift alternatives. For the primary modification, a lifter simply needs access to a weight belt and two stable elevation platforms for the feet (anything over a foot in height should be sufficient).

For reference, a weight belt is not the same as a lifting belt; the two are often confused. A lifting belt, mentioned in chapter 5, is used to stabilize the spine and can be adjusted for tightness. The support and added stability it provides can improve performance and safety in lifts like squats, deadlifts, overhead presses, and the Olympic lifts. A weight belt strictly serves one purpose: to add external loading to a typically unloaded exercise (like parallel bar dips). Using it strategically to replace a hip belt machine can be a useful purpose for it.

Loading the weight belt with plates or kettlebells and standing on the platforms above the ground is the way to perform this exercise with full range of motion (figure 6.10a). As a side note, the number of plates attached to the weight belt should be kept as minimal as possible. Loading four 25-pound (12 kg) plates instead of

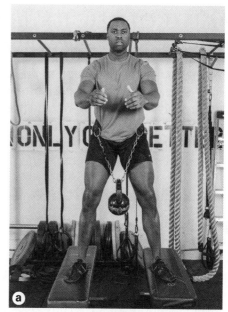

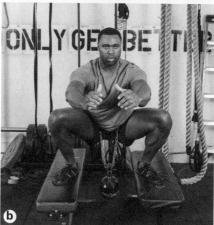

FIGURE 6.10 Weight belt squat: start position *(a)*, and finish *(b)*.

two 45-pound (20 kg) plates, just as an example, will mean twice the width occupying the space between the legs, which may get cumbersome. Since this movement is indeed a makeshift hack, it's understandable that there will be other factors to consider, such as the amount of weight being limited in the big picture (it's tough to load much more than 150 pounds [70 kg]), and it's also worth considering that a lifter will need to account for a mild swing factor with the weight hanging between the legs, rather than attached to a plate-loaded machine (figure 6.10b). This is not the lift variation for chasing major strength gains, and like its machine-based counterpart, it should be used as an accessory movement for higher reps.

Tall Lifters, Lifters With Long Legs and Long Femurs, and Posterior Chain Emphasis

The fact that these groups of people will need plenty of forward shin angle for a successful squat undoubtedly means the quads will be at work even more than for an average-built lifter. It can be frustrating if one goal of using the squat pattern is to develop the hamstrings and glutes. It's for these reasons the squat in its basic forms (front or back, full range of motion) probably isn't the best fit for these lifters.

Box Squat With a Lower Bar Position

Using the box squat coupled with a lower bar position can allow the shins to remain more vertical while the lifter reaches back farther with the hips to take a tight seat on the middle of the box. The box should not be at a lifter's full depth, but rather somewhere around a parallel upper thigh angle to ensure that anterior pelvic tilt isn't lost (figure 6.11a). This will keep the hamstring group taut and not forfeit any work the hip extensors need to contribute, and it will increase the amount of power and force output needed by the active muscles in order to perform the lift (McBride et al. 2010).

We recommend wearing flat shoes for box squatting, rather than Olympic lifting shoes, to ensure a more vertical shin position. Moreover, the seat taken on the box cannot be lax. The muscles must retain full tension through the entire movement (figure 6.11b). Enough weight should be placed on the box

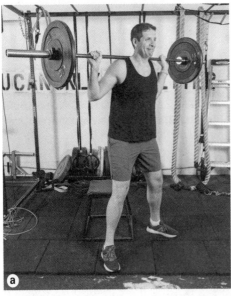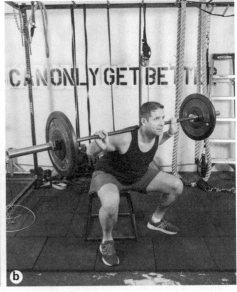

FIGURE 6.11   Box squat: start position *(a)*, and finish *(b)*.

for a seat to be taken and momentum to be removed from the equation, but not so much weight that the spine loses its positioning. Using a slightly wider stance with the feet and knees can help with posterior chain activity during this pattern and also help incorporate the inner thigh musculature a bit more.

Free Barbell Squat to Parallel Depth

Alternating weeks of the box squat with a free barbell squat to parallel depth with no pause can be a useful programming choice to engage the same muscle groups and still emphasize the posterior chain, while making use of the stretch–shortening cycle that was eliminated from the picture in the box squat. Any loading variation for parallel squats can work, including safety bars, barbells, or single dumbbells or kettlebells. If the goal is strength, both of these variations can and should be loaded fairly heavy, while still respecting the knee joints' comfort level. Once again, these squats are best performed with flat shoes, rather than shoes that have a distinct heel wedge, in order to maintain a more vertical shin angle.

Removing the body's ability to squat deep by choice also removes the reliance on the knee extensors, or quadriceps. However, during deep squat sessions, tactically using static stretching can be an effective strategy. Static stretching can temporarily impair neurological involvement of a muscle and ultimately weaken it for a brief period. A lifter can use that notion to their advantage when looking for more glute or hamstring activity in a squat pattern. Between sets of a squat, spending the majority of the rest time in a static stretch for the quads and hips can force them to be less involved in moving the load, shifting more of that responsibility toward the other players—like the glutes and hamstrings—to pick up the slack. This way, even during normal squatting workouts, a lifter can make the most out of the work the posterior chain is asked to do.

Squat Loading for Lifters With Bad Knees

The deadlift is a pulling exercise, and as such, it places little impact on the joints of the lower body. Rarely have we encountered a client complaining of knee stress from deadlifting, a posterior chain–based movement. Plus, the deadlift requires a shin angle that's nearly vertical, meaning zero knee-over-toe positioning to rely largely on the knee extensors and joint capsule. Squatting, on the other hand, is a pushing exercise. That means the forces are coming down directly on the joints, and it's the body's responsibility to press up *under* that weight. For most lifters who suffer from poor knee health, this spells trouble when it comes to virtually any squat variation. We've found that not only previously injured lifters but also tall and long-legged lifters and ectomorph body types tend to have a history of chronic or acute knee pain that is exacerbated during squats—even with good technique. The reason is the shin angle these squatters need in order to achieve a deep squat (and the stress forces on the knee joint that come along with that). Any differences in strength between the anterior and posterior chain muscles can worsen the situation as far as discomfort endured, since each muscle in the complex isn't doing everything it can to contribute.

Deeper degrees of flexion, accompanied by greater anterior translation of the knee, are usually more demanding on the connective tissue of the joint, and bearing load at bottom end ranges requires plenty of torque to be produced to exit these positions. To make squatting possible for these individuals who do indeed require a deeper shin angle, it's worth taking a closer look at the resistance profile chosen for the pattern. A resistance profile (or resistance curve) can often be confused for a lifter's strength (or force) curve, though the two should not be used interchangeably. A strength, or force, curve refers to the output a given muscle can provide through each phase of a rep. However, a resistance curve describes the nature of what the lifter is lifting. A dumbbell biceps curl done normally, for instance, will have portions within that movement where the weight will load the working muscle more and be more difficult to lift, as well as portions within the movement where the weight will not load the working muscle quite as much and be easier to maneuver. Changing the implement from a dumbbell to a band, kettlebell, or chain will significantly change the resistance curve of the exercise, despite the movement pattern itself being exactly the same.

Lifting With Chain or Band Resistance

Attaching chains to the barbell, or bands (wrapped around the barbell and anchored to the floor), is a way to manipulate the resistance profile (figure 6.12*a-b*). Since the joints are a bit more vulnerable in the bottom position

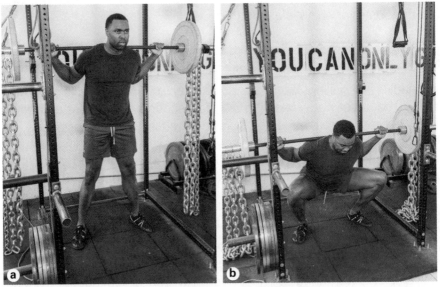

FIGURE 6.12   Chain squat: start position *(a)*, and finish *(b)*.

of a squat, having the majority of the chain's links on the ground while at the bottom makes the weight the body has to bear lighter (compared with the top of the lift, when more links come off the ground). Likewise, the band tension at the bottom of a squat will be lesser than the tension at the top (figure 6.13). This is an intelligent way to expose the nervous system to a resistance that rivals a lifter's best efforts while protecting the joints from that high load at the bottom of each rep. Cumulatively speaking, it can be a major difference maker for the health and overall wellness of the joints—especially the knees.

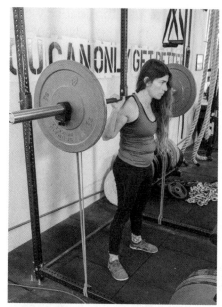

FIGURE 6.13 Banded squat setup.

Lifting With a Band Target

Creating some assistance through difficult portions of a heavy lift is not easy. Lifters most commonly rely on a reverse band setup. Bands are looped around the top of a power cage and come down around the barbell. When applied to a loaded bar, the bands are the most stretched—and ultimately provide the most assistance—through the bottom end range of the lift, where the bar is closest to the ground. As the weight ascends, the bar receives less assistance as the tension decreases in the bands. The problem is, it isn't possible to set this up in many gyms, because of either the overall difficulty of doing so or (more commonly) the lack of proper equipment. For example, power racks (figure 6.14a) differ from squat cages (figure 6.14b) in that they have no overhead bars from which bands can be hung, voiding the reverse band idea to break plateaus or save joints. With these restrictions understood, it's worth getting creative to produce a similar effect.

The band target squat can be a game changer for lifters who are looking to gain strength. It not only provides assistance at the bottom end but also builds confidence thanks to the tactile cue it can give an individual during a set. If a lifter struggles with depth issues, this can also provide some consistency under heavy loads.

A tight band across the safety pins, set at a lifter's desired height, will gently sling the lifter out of the bottom position and take pressure off the knees while in that position, which is perfect for people suffering from joint discomfort (including the knee joint) during loaded movement. The beauty of this hack is that if you need more help, you just add more bands. This can create just the kinetic edge needed to get a heavy weight out of the hole and still deal with the entire load for the majority of the rep, including the lockout.

Taking advantage of this hack, especially during heavier sets, can be just what the doctor ordered. To do this exercise properly, a lifter would set up a barbell back or front squat in the rack the normal way and set the safety pins at a height that's between 6 and 12 inches (15-30 cm) above the lifter's bottom depth (using the buttocks as frame of reference).

Stretch a band or bands across the pins, and make sure they're pulled tight and flat. Pay attention to their placement, and ensure they're in line with the lifter's lower glutes at the bottom of the squat. Too far forward and they won't help. Too far backward and the lifter may miss them entirely.

The lifter will then unrack the weight and step back until about 4 to 6 inches (10-15 cm) in front of the band (figure 6.15a). The next step is to squat to full range, establishing good contact on the band

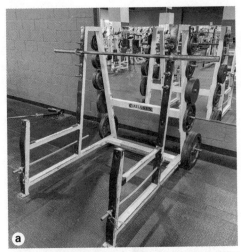

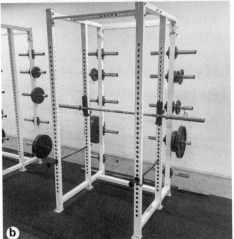

FIGURE 6.14 Power rack (a), and squat cage (b).

with the glutes. The lifter lets the band help the initiation of the concentric rep while maintaining good form (figure 6.15b). Focus on low reps per set; three to six is a smart range.

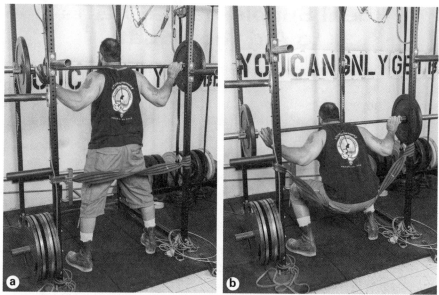

FIGURE 6.15 Band target squat: start position *(a)*, and finish *(b)*.

Knee Sleeves

Lastly, wrapping the knees by wearing sleeves can help in the same way a belt can benefit a lifter's spine. The compression that knee wraps provide stabilizes the joint, instills confidence in the lifter, and even helps sling the lifter out of the bottom position, thanks to the tension on the threads a very stretched sleeve can create in positions of deep flexion. In our experience, very few lifters say squatting with knee sleeves makes the knees feel worse than squatting without them. Especially if the plan for the day is to squat heavy weight, they're a worthwhile investment. Even the simple Tensor sleeves available at a local pharmacy can provide the support needed, but strength training–specific stores carry more performance-oriented sleeves that are thicker and more durable. A lifter needs to choose the best fit for them.

Ideal Supplementary Lifts to Aid the Squat

The movements to supplement a lifting pattern might not be identical, but they still have carryover. Nothing will make squatting stronger more than practicing the squat itself, but some movements can significantly affect knee and hip extension and are suitable for all body types to bolster lifting strength and skill:

- Leg press (especially important for big lifters)
- Walking lunge
- Rear-foot-elevated split squat
- Leg extension
- Leg curl (we especially like using the prone leg curl as a pre-exhaust method to warm up the knee joint from the posterior side; starting a squat workout with three or four sets of leg curls always results in a happier squat session)

Of all the lift patterns included in this book, the squat pattern is arguably the most contentious. Different schools of thought and coaching methods can cause a world of disagreement beyond the key principles of the movement. Here, we've played the safe route by breaking down anthropometric differences that can prevent those principles from being respected, while leaving enough of this information up to the reader to decide just how to apply it to things like foot width, depth, and foot angle. This entire book is based around the notion of saying goodbye to blanket cues and rules surrounding popular lifts, and as such, it's very much in keeping with the theme to depart from those strictures, especially during a movement like the squat.

Chapter 7

The Bench Press

We talked in depth about basic bench press form in chapter 3. There is one point, however, that deserves some elaboration. The bench press is a horizontal press from the chest area toward the ceiling. One would assume that a straight line, being the shortest distance from the start of the press to the finish, would therefore be ideal for the bench press. And while this is, in theory, true—a curved path elongates the time the bar is being pressed, and therefore will increase the amount of metabolic work required to complete the press—the ideal path of the bar will tend to be slightly curved. The nature of the curve is determined by the structure of the shoulder as well as the leg drive of the press. The arch of the spine combined with the leg drive force the bar to travel toward the head a bit before the body's mechanics are in an optimal position to press the bar straight up. The flatter the back of the lifter and the less leg drive used, the less of a J curve there tends to be.

Although lever positioning is important, just as important is the ability to optimally apply force through that lever. An extra-wide bench press, for example, while providing the advantage of a shorter bar path, may not be ideal for lifters who cannot apply appropriate force through that particular lever setup. The needs and preferences of the individual should always be prioritized over the physics of the lift.

The Perfect Bench Press Body Type

The bodies that are best suited to bench pressing are those that create an environment in which the bar travels the shortest distance. Therefore, lifters with short arms (short; short arms and long legs; short torso, long legs, and short arms) and lifters with large bodies (big all over) generally prevail in the bench press. Alternatively, a lifter who is capable of a tremendous spinal arch can also drastically reduce the length of the path of the barbell, mimicking the advantage of the lifter with a large torso.

Leg length doesn't come into play much here—if the lifter's legs are too short to make appropriate contact with the floor, the lifter can simply press the feet against platforms. While the bench press does not require much grip capacity, hand size may play a role in that a smaller hand may be more conducive to positioning the bar above the wrist rather than farther back on the hand. The straighter the wrist, and the more in line with the wrist the barbell can be placed, the stronger the bench press will be.

Studies on advanced lifters (mainly powerlifters) did not find a significant correlation between arm length and bench press strength (Keogh et al. 2005). However, in these cases, any disadvantage of arm length may have been offset by a larger arm circumference. While longer arms mean more distance for the barbell to travel, they also mean a greater area for muscle tissue to grow (Caruso et al. 2012). Heavily muscled lifters tend to have higher 1RMs in bench press whether they have long arms or not. Ultimately, bigger lifters seem to bench best, regardless of limb length. That said, there may be a stronger correlation between longer arm length and greater fatigue in the bench press, resulting in reduced performance (Bellar et al. 2010).

Bench Press: Long Arms

The most obvious issue with having long arms in the bench press is that the bar has to be pressed a much longer distance. This does not seem to affect the mechanics of the lift, but it does mean the athlete must perform more work to press the barbell (Lockie et al. 2018). Because the lifter is expending more energy in the lift than might a shorter-armed athlete, the risk of fatigue is higher. This can be somewhat reconciled if the lifter has

1. a flexible enough back to create a very prominent arch and
2. a large enough torso to make up for a major portion of the distance the bar would need to travel.

A long-armed lifter's bench press also has a larger amount of torque—the bar sits farther from the fulcrums (i.e., the glenohumeral and elbow joints), which means the muscles around those joints must produce more force in order to move the bar. The lengths of the segments also matter here—a shorter or longer-than-average humerus, for instance, will change the amount of torque on the elbow and glenohumeral joints.

Tips for the Long-Armed Lifter

A short torso could put the long-armed lifter at a particular disadvantage because the degree of the lifter's arch would be limited by the length of the torso. The following suggestions are useful additions to the arsenal of any long-armed lifter, and in particular lifters with both long arms and short torsos.

Tuck the Feet

By pulling the feet behind the body, the lifter will naturally increase the arch in their back (figure 7.1). Even if the lifter is not particularly flexible, any extra height here can increase the amount of weight able to be lifted in the bench press. Some leg drive will be lost as a result, but the shortening of the bar path will be beneficial.

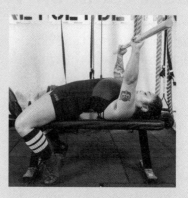

Figure 7.1   Barbell bench press with tucked feet.

Use a Wide Grip

Having an extremely wide bench press is one way to address how far the bar needs to be pressed, but as discussed earlier, an extra-wide bench press may not be the strongest press for many people. Furthermore, there are limits to the width of the grip in powerlifting competitions, so if an athlete plans to compete, they will not have the option of placing their arms wider than what is allowed. However, taking a slightly wider than shoulder-width grip, or going to the limits of what the lifting federation allows (if the lifter is a competitor), will help shorten the distance of the press.

A wide-grip bench press may put the shoulder at greater risk of injury, particularly on the descent of the barbell, because of the amount of external rotation and abduction of the shoulder in this position (Green and Comfort 2007). The risk of injury increases as the hands extend to and beyond 1.5 times the width of the shoulders. If an athlete has pain or discomfort in this position, a narrower grip may be advised.

Train the Bar Path

The long-armed lifter in particular needs to be consistent with where the bar is placed on the chest at the bottom of the lift and the ideal bar path that is strongest for that lifter. Any area beyond the highest point on the body when the body is in bench press position will further increase the distance the bar needs to be pressed, so every fraction of an inch counts. It is a good strategy to bench-press multiple times per week in order to maximize strength gains in the lift; in this way, an appropriate training volume can be achieved fairly easily (Grgic et al. 2018). At each training session, the lifter should focus on exactly where the bar should land on the chest, as well as solidifying the J shape of the press.

Because of the longer bar path, longer-armed lifters must generate a lot of power off the chest to gain enough momentum to carry the press through the whole range of motion without fatiguing. They also need to focus on strengthening the sticking points of the lift to keep the bar from stalling before lockout. Several variations of the bench press can assist in these areas.

Best Variation: Pin Press

Another exercise that will increase strength and endurance in the upper portion of the bench press is the pin press. The setup is much like the bench press, but the pins or safety bars are set up in the rack at about 3 to 5 inches (8-13 cm) directly above the spot on the chest where the bar would normally land (figure 7.2a). Because the bar comes to a dead stop at the pins, the lifter will need to generate force without the benefit of the stretch reflex that helps drive the press off the chest (figure 7.2b). This will strengthen the lift in an area where form is more likely to break down. The pin press also strengthens the triceps, which is particularly important for those with longer arms.

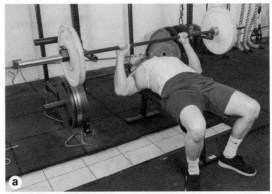
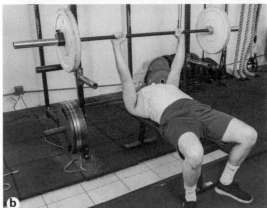

FIGURE 7.2 Pin press: start position (a), and finish (b).

Floor Press

If the lifter is not a competitive athlete, there might not be a reason to bench-press from the bench. Floor presses are easier on the shoulder joint and provide a much more manageable range of motion for the bar to move through. Furthermore, the long-armed lifter is likely to fatigue in the latter portion of the lift. Training in that range of motion can help increase strength and muscular endurance in that range.

The floor press is performed similarly to the bench press, except the lifter lies supine on the floor rather than on a bench, feet flat on the floor, knees bent (figure 7.3a). The path of the elbows is limited by the floor, so

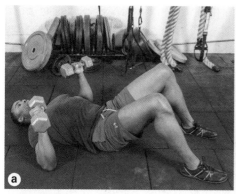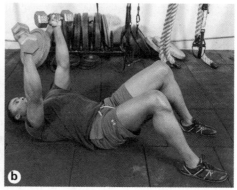

FIGURE 7.3   Floor press: start position *(a)*, and finish *(b)*.

this movement is a partial bench press. The other main difference between the floor press and the bench press is there is no leg drive in the floor press, so the lift is purely driven by the upper body (figure 7.3*b*). There is no real requirement for leg positioning in this movement; some lifters prefer to have their legs positioned straight out in front of them, and some prefer a bent knee position with feet flat on the floor. The leg positioning will generally not affect the quality of the floor press.

Chains and Bands

Adding chains or elastic bands to the bench press is another way to increase strength at the top end (figure 7.4). The lifter is still able to generate a great deal of power off the chest in these lifts because the barbell is lightest at the bottom. As more of the chains come off the floor, or as the bands are stretched farther, the barbell becomes heavier. These movements are useful

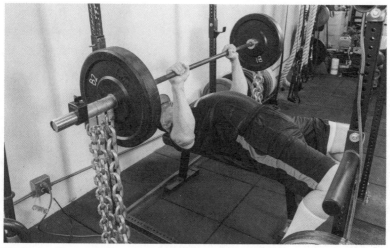

FIGURE 7.4   Chain press.

for increasing the ability to produce as much momentum as possible from the chest to work through sticking points, as well as providing neurological feedback from holding a heavier-than-usual weight at lockout.

Board Press

The board press is another method long-armed lifters can use to strengthen the movement through their sticking points without the benefit of the initial stretch at the bottom of the lift. It is performed similarly to the bench press, but boards of desired thickness are placed in the middle of the chest (figure 7.5a). The bar will touch the boards instead of the chest, thus shortening the bar path (figure 7.5b). Boards are often made with a handle at the bottom, like a paddle, so that a training partner can hold them steady on the lifter's chest; this is one of the safest ways to perform a board press, because an unsecured board can slip. There are also products that attach directly to the handle of the bar to create the same effect as a board, providing a safer option for lifters training alone.

While there is no standard board width, most boards are somewhere between 1 and 2 inches (3-5 cm) and can be stacked as necessary. The athlete can use any number of boards to train specific ranges of the press. The lifter must first recognize the ranges in which they are weakest and then use the appropriate number of blocks to specifically train in that range of motion and increase strength through that sticking point. Training these partial ranges of motion is a way to increase training volume without overstressing the shoulders. Volume training can help increase not only strength but also muscle hypertrophy, and, as we discuss earlier in this chapter, more mass leads to better bench presses.

In partial presses such as the board press, the lifter can lift heavier loads than they might be able to in a full range of motion press. The boards can

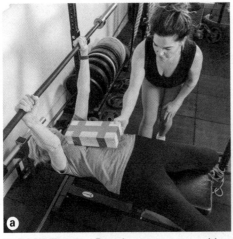
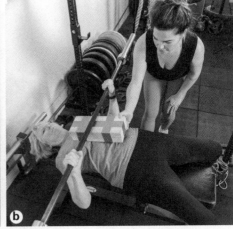

FIGURE 7.5   Board press: start position *(a)*, and finish *(b)*.

also be used to continue work with the same weight after the full range of motion press is fatigued, therefore allowing more volume of training within the same workout.

Reverse Banded Bench Press

In the reverse banded bench press, it is best to use a power rack and long, loop-style bands. Put one end of the loop over the middle of the top of the power rack, in the position directly above where the barbell will be when the athlete is pressing. Pull the rest of the band through the loop so that the band is secured at the top of the rack (figure 7.6a). Do the same with the other band on the other side of the power rack. Be sure the two bands are as evenly tensioned as possible so they provide the same amount of resistance on each side of the barbell.

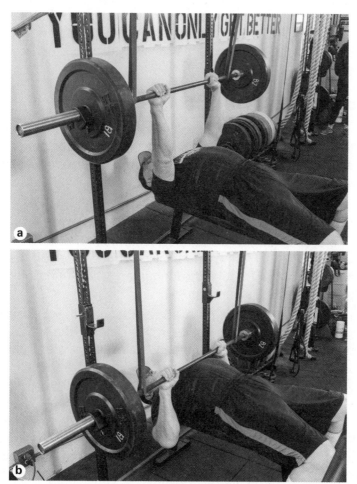

FIGURE 7.6   Reverse banded press: start position *(a)*, and finish *(b)*.

Loop the free end of the bands around the barbell on whichever side of the plates the athlete prefers, as long as the bands are evenly placed on the bar. Test the press a few times before using the working weight—if the bands are pulling the bar off track, they will need to be adjusted so they are directly in line with the bar path (figure 7.6*b*).

Attaching stretch bands to the top of a power rack as opposed to the bottom provides the opposite stimulus of a traditional banded bench press in which the bands are affixed to the bottom of the rack. In this method, the bands support a portion of the barbell's weight at the chest, and as the bar is pressed, it becomes heavier as the stretch is taken out of the bands. The amount of assistance provided by the bands depends on the thickness and age of the bands as well as the height of the rack to which they are attached.

This is another method longer-armed lifters can use to more safely overload a press, locking out a heavier weight than they could normally press from full range of motion. It is also a good way to generate more force through the sticking points of a press, much in the way as adding chains or bands to the bottom of the press. With chains or bands, the lifter can produce more force in the top of the lift with a heavier weight than otherwise possible (Swinton et al. 2011).

1.5-Repetition Bench Press

In the 1.5-repetition bench press, the lifter presses the bar halfway up, then returns it to the chest and performs a full-repetition bench press. The long-armed lifter in particular may benefit from this combination of partial- and full-range bench press for a few reasons:

1. The lifter will get extra lifting volume from the chest to about the sticking point in every lift. Training this portion of the bench press can increase strength in that specific range of motion (Newmire and Willoughby 2018). Having a particularly strong press off the chest will help propel the bar through the longer range of motion inherent in the long-armed athlete's bench press.

2. The extra volume within each 1.5 repetitions can increase muscular endurance. As discussed earlier in this chapter, the long-armed lifter is more likely to fatigue in the bench press because of the distance the barbell needs to be pressed. The 1.5-repetition bench press is an excellent way to increase volume within a movement.

3. Combining partial range of motion lifts with full range of motion lifts has the potential to maximize muscle hypertrophy (Newmire and Willoughby 2018). You have learned in this chapter that a larger arm circumference and a larger body circumference are important for optimal bench press strength. The 1.5-repetition bench press is one mechanism that can be used to achieve more muscle mass.

Triceps Strengthening

The placement of the long-armed lifter's hands on the bar in relation to their shoulders will result in a narrower grip than that of a shorter-armed lifter in the same hand position. Therefore, the long-armed lifter will likely need to generate more force from their triceps to press the bar off the chest than would the shorter-armed lifter, because the angle between the arms and torso will likely be smaller at the bottom of the lift. Movements that strengthen the triceps should be prominent in a long-armed lifter's programming. We discuss accessory movements for the bench press in chapter 12. The Tate press, in particular, is a triceps exercise that specifically pertains to the bench press.

Close-Grip Bench Press

The mechanics of the close-grip bench press are more or less the same as that of the traditional bench press. The hands are placed at or slightly narrower than the width of the shoulders (figure 7.7a), or at approximately 16 inches (40 cm) apart (Lockie and Moreno 2017). Bench pressing with a narrower grip increases shoulder abduction (Lockie and Moreno 2017). This can help reduce the tendency to flare the elbows, a common issue when the lifter's triceps are weaker (figure 7.7b). The narrower, elbows-in position can also take stress off the shoulders (Lockie and Moreno 2017). Since a longer-armed lifter may have more stress at the bottom of the shoulder

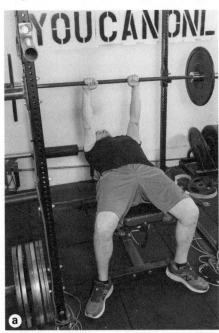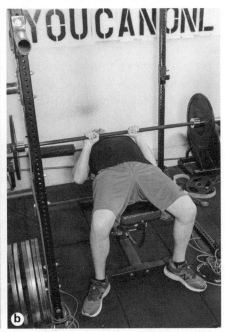

FIGURE 7.7 Close-grip press: start position *(a)*, and finish *(b)*.

because of greater stretching of the pectoral and anterior deltoid muscles in that position as compared with a shorter-armed lifter, adding close-grip presses can be an excellent way to increase pressing volume with lower risk of injury.

The close-grip press increases the activity of the triceps brachii and decreases the activity of the sternoclavicular portion of the pectoralis major (Lehman 2005). While all bench press grip widths recruit the triceps, the narrow grip in particular is a useful tool for strengthening the triceps. Because the triceps brachii is responsible for straightening the arm at the elbow, the close-grip bench press can help the athlete obtain a more powerful lockout at the top of the press.

Incline Bench Press

When the bench is angled for an incline bench press, the size of the torso may play a lesser role unless the lifter has significant girth in the upper portion of the pectorals. The incline bench press can be an excellent addition to a bench press program, allowing for more recruitment of the anterior deltoid and upper pectoral fibers (Rodríguez-Ridao, D., et al, 2020) and providing an alternative to training the flat bench press to help limit repetitive stress injury risk (figure 7.8a-b).

To perform the incline bench press, the lifter should first choose the angle at which they would like to train. A bench angle of approximately 30 degrees will place more emphasis on the upper pectoral region, while a bench angle of 45 degrees or more will train the anterior deltoids more and reduce activation of pectoralis major (Rodríguez-Ridao, D., et al, 2020). Once the lifter has chosen their bench angle, the lifter will position themselves underneath the bar and choose their desired grip width. For most lifters, holding the bar slightly wider than shoulder width will suffice; wide grip and narrow grip incline bench press can be utilized as well much in the same way and for the same reasons that they would be performed for flat bench press. For a standard incline bench press, the forearms will ideally be perpendicular to the floor. The feet will be flat on the floor, knees placed in line with the ankles.

The lifter will place the head, upper back, and hips on the bench, unrack the barbell and stabilize it with arms perpendicular to the floor and elbows in a locked position. Pulling the shoulder blades down and back in the same manner in which a flat bench press is performed will help put the shoulders in a better pressing position and will help stabilize the weight. The lifter will then actively pull the barbell to the chest while maintaining the "open" position of the chest and shoulders. It may help to think about pulling the elbows towards each other at the bottom of the lift. Once the barbell touches the upper chest, the lifter will push the feet into the floor without raising the body off the bench seat, and will press the barbell off the chest and back to the start position, taking care not to flare the elbows.

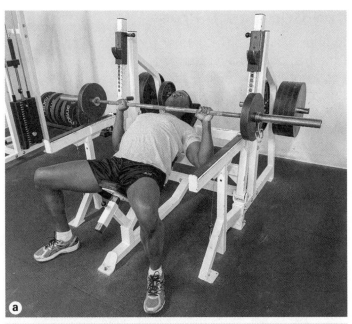

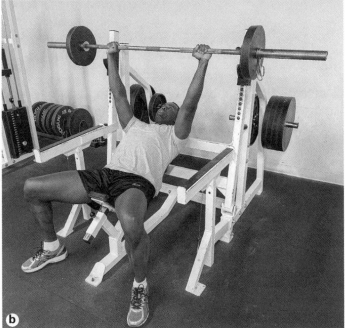

FIGURE 7.8 Incline bench press: start position *(a)*, and finish *(b)*.

The incline bench press can be performed with dumbbells or kettlebells as well, which provide a similar benefit to a dumbbell or kettlebell bench press. The lift can be performed unilaterally as well, if desired, which will force the lifter to stabilize their body against the uneven weight.

Supinated-Grip Bench Press

Should the lifter wish to have greater recruitment of the sternoclavicular portion of the pectoralis major, they can rotate the palms so their thumbs face each other on the bar (figure 7.9). This grip maintains the recruitment of the triceps brachii and also keeps the activation of the pectoralis major (Lehman 2005). In addition, this particular grip provides significant biceps brachii recruitment, which can help stabilize the shoulders more.

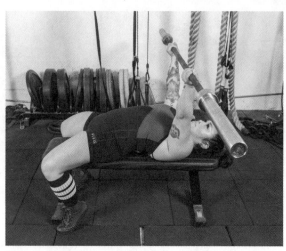

FIGURE 7.9   Barbell bench press with supinated grip.

The supinated grip keeps the elbows from flaring and may produce a more comfortable lift for athletes with shoulder injuries. It may also strengthen the wrists, which is key in maintaining proper barbell placement. However, this particular lift tends to land lower on the body and does not follow the same J-shaped path as a traditional bench press. It is therefore not ideal for practicing bench press technique, but it offers an alternative pressing movement where needed or desired.

While long arms and a shorter torso may provide challenges for the bench press, proper programming and positioning can greatly improve performance in this lift. If bench pressing proves problematic, and should a conventional bench press not be imperative for the athlete, many of the previous suggestions offer similar benefits.

Bench Press: Short Arms; Large Bodies

Short-armed and large-bodied athletes tend to excel at the bench press, since their bench press path will be shortest. It may be useful, however, to find extra challenges for the short-armed lifter to create a greater training effect. Exercises that reduce the efficiency of the lift, like the paused press, or increase the range of motion of the press, like the dumbbell or cambered bar bench press, can help even the most ideal bench press athlete improve the lift even more.

Best Variation: Dumbbell or Kettlebell Bench Press

Using dumbbells or kettlebells for the bench press exercise is another way the longer-armed lifter can gain strength at the bottom of the lift. This is also an excellent way for a lifter with shorter arms or a large torso to achieve a greater range of motion than what their levers typically allow in a barbell press.

Dumbbells and kettlebells allow the weights to be lowered past the limits of the chest so that a greater range of motion can be trained (figure 7.10*a*). Dumbbell or kettlebell pressing also allows for more freedom of arm placement throughout the movement, therefore making the lift potentially more comfortable than barbell pressing for athletes with shoulder pain. Both arms must provide equal force to lift the weights, and so this can be one way of reducing strength discrepancies between the arms (figure 7.10*b*).

When a lifter is holding a kettlebell in a press position, the wrist must remain completely straight. Because the kettlebell sits on the back of the arm, providing resistance to the straight wrist position, it stands to reason that using a kettlebell for the bench press might benefit the strength of the wrist flexors. This can lead to better positioning of the barbell in the press.

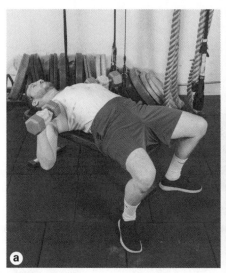 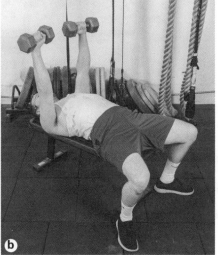

FIGURE 7.10   Dumbbell bench press: start position *(a)*, and finish *(b)*.

Paused Bench Press

Pausing the bar for a few seconds at the bottom of the bench press has a few benefits. First of all, it allows the lifter to gain consistency in exactly where on the chest the bar lands. As we discuss earlier, for long-armed lifters in particular, ensuring that the bar touches precisely the right spot on the body can make a tremendous difference in how much weight is able to be pressed. For lifters with short arms or big torsos, the reduced efficiency of the paused press makes it significantly more challenging, and therefore it can improve overall bench press performance.

The paused bench press also prevents the lifter from bouncing the bar off the chest, a common cheat used to propel the bar back up. This also means the lifter is forced to have better control over the lowering portion of the lift, reducing risk of injury and increasing bar path accuracy.

Cambered Bar

Using a cambered or bowed bar is another way an athlete can increase bench press strength in a greater range of motion than a traditional barbell allows. Use of the cambered bar (figure 7.11) in training has been demonstrated to increase bar velocity and power output in the bench press (Krysztofik et al. 2020). The cambered bar makes good use of the stretch–shortening cycle to help propel the bar higher, thus making it ideal for the long-armed lifter. This is also another excellent tool to help lifters with short arms or large torsos extend their range of motion in the bench press.

Because the cambered bar places the shoulders at a greater stretch at the bottom of the lift, it may put the shoulders at a higher risk of injury. Avoid this, or any, movement if the athlete experiences pain from its use.

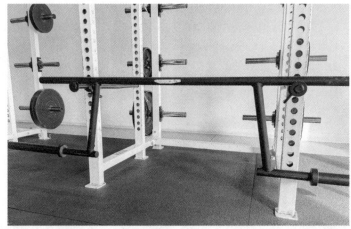

FIGURE 7.11   Cambered bar.

Hand Size and Bench Pressing

Because a larger hand allows for more surface area for the bar to potentially inhabit, it may be more challenging for a lifter with bigger hands to properly place the barbell over the wrist in the bench press. Proper positioning of the barbell is important not only for a stronger press but also for reducing risk of injury. A wrist out of alignment could also mean an elbow in a problematic position, which can also negatively affect the shoulder.

Wrist wraps are widely used in competitive powerlifting events and may be useful for those lifters who have difficulty achieving a straight wrist position with a barbell. Wraps can help stabilize the wrist and prevent it from falling too far into extension. Strengthening the wrist flexors is important for proper barbell positioning. We discuss forearm strengthening movements for this purpose in chapter 12.

Hooked Acromion Process and Bench Pressing

The bench press might be especially uncomfortable for an athlete with a type III (hooked) acromion process, regardless of arm length (figure 7.12*a-b*). This type of bone structure is commonly associated with shoulder impingement and bursitis and can be a cause of full rotator cuff tears (Inklebarger et al. 2017). The eccentric portion of the lift might be of particular discomfort. In the case of this type of morphology, or of any pain with pressing, it may be best to stick with other, nonpainful movements that train the pectoral region. If bench pressing causes pain, and if this lift is not imperative for the athlete, providing alternative movements may be the best course of action. Push-ups, chest flys, cable crossovers, or any other movements that do not exacerbate the individual's injuries may be used. Possible movements are described in chapter 12. Another bench press alternative that might be of use is the dumbbell or kettlebell bench press, as described earlier in this chapter.

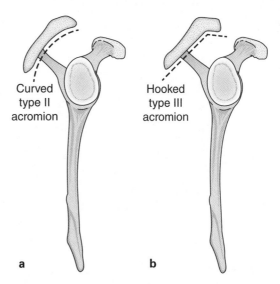

FIGURE 7.12 Type II (normal) acromion process *(a)*, and Type III (hooked) acromion process *(b)*.

Using a Multigrip Bar

A multigrip barbell can provide variation in the bench press, and it also has a number of sport-specific uses (figure 7.13). Lifters with long arms or with shoulder pain may find that a neutral grip or an angled grip provides a more comfortable position from which to press. A multigrip bar allows for positioning

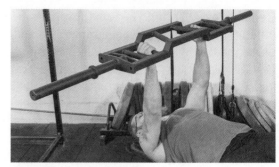

FIGURE 7.13   Multigrip barbell.

in which the elbows remain closer to the body, reducing the risk of injury associated with elbow flaring.

While having a body type that makes the barbell have to travel a longer way can be a big disadvantage in pressing movements, there are a number of ways an athlete can compensate for this. From changing the position of the body (increasing the arch height, for instance) to the dimensions of the body (e.g., putting on more muscle mass or torso circumference) to focusing on getting stronger through sticking points, bench press performance can be improved exponentially in many ways. Even for those athletes who simply struggle with the bench press in any circumstance, this compound movement is well worth practicing because it is an excellent way to build upper body mass and horizontal pushing strength.

Chapter 8

The Overhead Press

Most of the research on anthropometry has centered around the bench press. The few existing studies, to our knowledge, that examine the relationship between body segment lengths and overhead work use the Olympic lifts (the snatch and the clean and jerk) as their subject movements. The studies performed on overhead athletes so far have very small subject pools, and therefore a great deal more research is needed to make more solid conclusions about the relationship between anthropometrics and vertical pressing exercises. That said, based on the available research, the current knowledge of biomechanics, and our own experience as coaches, there does appear to be some overlap between the kinematics of the vertical and horizontal pressing movements and anthropometry.

The Perfect Overhead Press Body Type

Much like the bench press, athletes with greater muscle mass seem to perform best in vertical pressing movements (Pérez et al. 2021). While a larger torso is useful in the bench press, regardless of body composition, Pérez and colleagues found that, at least for Olympic athletes, more lean body mass and less fat mass are important for the overhead lifts. This brings us to two possible ideal body types for overhead lifting:

1. According to Pérez, shorter limb length provides the best mechanical advantage for a stronger lift, pound for pound.
2. However, longer limbs provide a bigger surface area, and therefore a superior landscape for building more muscle mass.

Therefore, the ideal body type for the vertical press could be either a shorter-limbed athlete or a longer-limbed athlete. Either way, the ideal pressing method will be different depending on the body type of the lifter.

The overhead press is an excellent test of upper body strength and overall strength and stability, so it is definitely a valuable lift for any body type. The following suggestions can make overhead pressing more accessible for body types that may have more trouble with a traditional barbell military press.

Overhead Press: Long Forearms

Regardless of the length of the limbs, a lifter with longer forearms relative to total arm length will be at an initial disadvantage in the overhead press. In the rack position, the barbell will ideally sit on top of the fronts of the shoulders. However, a longer forearm will cause the bar to sit higher than the deltoids, and therefore it will not rack optimally (figure 8.1). This position can be problematic for some because any leg drive used in the press might not transfer well to the lift owing to the disconnect between the body and the bar.

When the upper arm is shorter in comparison to the forearm, the lifter might try to force the barbell into position by pulling the elbows backward. This would put the forearm at an awkward angle, making it difficult to transfer force upward in an efficient way. The ideal position of the forearm in a press, as we discussed earlier in this book, is perpendicular to the floor, with the barbell resting on the lower portion of the palm directly above the wrist bones (figure 8.2). Any deviation from this position will result in a weaker, less powerful press. Here are two overhead press variations to optimize the lift for those with long forearms. These athletes will also benefit from the seated variations mentioned later in this chapter.

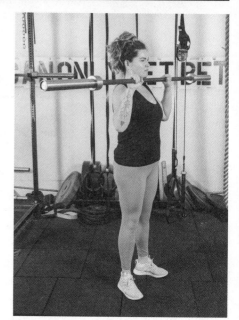

FIGURE 8.1   Rack position with long forearms.

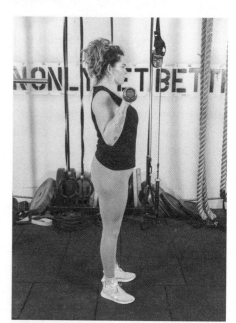

FIGURE 8.2   Ideal forearm position for barbell.

Best Variation: Strict Press

The strict press is simply a standing press in which there is absolutely no leg movement. The barbell starts in the racked position and is pressed straight overhead using the shoulders and arms alone. Because there is no leg drive in the strict press, it works well for lifters who cannot rest the bar properly on the shoulders, whether because of forearm length or poor flexibility in the upper body. The strict press is an excellent exercise for developing pure overhead press strength. While adding leg drive can increase the amount of weight able to be pressed overhead, the strict press challenges the strength of the upper body alone.

Landmine Press

The landmine press is ideal for lifters who cannot hold the barbell in the optimal rack position (figure 8.3a-b). It can also be a good movement for lifters with shoulder pain and an accessory movement to help train the overhead press at different angles. The landmine press can add volume to

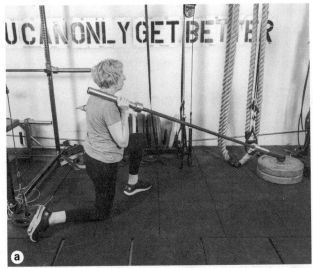

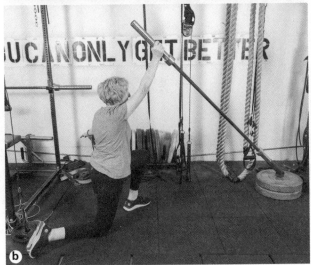

FIGURE 8.3   Landmine press: start position *(a)*, and finish *(b)*.

a pressing routine while reducing the risk of overuse injuries. The forearm is perpendicular to the line of the press, so this position is perfect for lifters who can't rack well with a perpendicular forearm.

Overhead Press: Long Torso

While the torso will move a bit in the initial portion of the overhead press, it is important not to exaggerate this backward movement. Relying too much on leaning backward in the overhead press is a very common error. Many lifters feel stronger in a more horizontal direction, or might not have the shoulder mobility to press straight overhead. Some lifters also lean backward because they fear hitting themselves in the face with the bar. However, leaning backward in the overhead press can put excessive strain on the lower back, and it increases the length of the bar path, making the press even more difficult. Individuals with longer torsos might find themselves at a particular risk of injury from leaning backward in the press, because the weight of the lift would be farther from the lower back than in a lifter with a shorter torso.

Best Variation: Seated Press

The seated press can be done with or without support for the torso. Either way, performing the press from the seated position reduces the tendency to lean backward (figure 8.4a). It also removes any leg drive, so, like the strict press, the work of the press is done completely by the upper body (figure

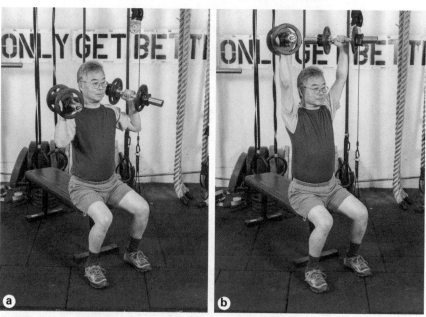

FIGURE 8.4   Seated press: start position *(a)*, and finish *(b)*.

8.4*b*). It therefore can be a useful lift for individuals with long forearms and others who cannot rack the barbell optimally on the deltoids.

Z Press

Like the seated press, the Z press removes leg drive and forces the torso to remain upright. The posterior chain is recruited significantly in the Z press, making it a good exercise for increasing shoulder stability. This can be useful not only for lifters with long torsos but also for those with longer arms (see more suggestions for long arms in the next section of this chapter).

The Z press requires the ability to remain seated bolt upright with the legs straight out in front (figure 8.5*a-b*). The lifter can modify this if needed by widening the legs so that the hips sit in a more comfortable position in the socket (figure 8.5*c*). It is also possible for the athlete to sit on a small step or platform to raise the hips a few inches should there be flexibility issues.

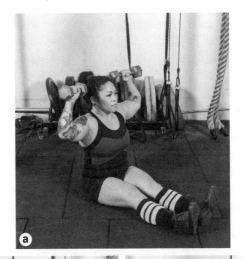

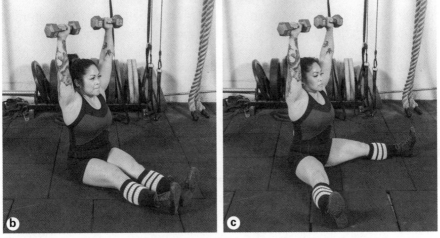

FIGURE 8.5 Z press: start position *(a)*, finish *(b)*, and modified stance *(c)*.

The seated press and Z press need to be done with a considerably lighter weight than a standing press because of the lack of leg drive, the narrower base of support, and the increased stability and flexibility requirements (particularly in the Z press).

Overhead Press: Long Arms

Much like the bench press, having long arms in the overhead press can be a disadvantage. The barbell has a longer path to travel, and fatigue can kick in more than it might for a lifter with shorter arms. Unlike the bench press, having a bigger torso will not change the distance the bar needs to travel—a longer-armed lifter simply has a longer range of motion than a shorter-armed athlete. Because the bar is farther from the shoulder joints and torso in the longer-armed athlete, stabilizing the bar may also be more challenging.

Improving the strength of the triceps, upper back, torso, and shoulder stabilizers will go a long way in increasing the strength and quality of the overhead press in long-armed athletes. We discuss specific accessory exercises to target these areas in chapter 12. Here are optimal variations of the overhead press.

Best Variation: Pin Press

The pin press in the overhead press has similar benefits to the pin press in the bench press mentioned in chapter 7—it helps strengthen the press through specific sticking points. Training the weakest points of the overhead press is valuable for any athlete, but because a longer-armed lifter is more likely to fatigue before lockout than a shorter-armed lifter, strength through sticking points is especially useful.

Pin placement will vary depending on the range of motion the lifter wants to train. If the athlete wants to work on lockout, for example, the pins should be placed above the halfway point of the press. If the lifter is more interested in training the midrange of the press, the pins can be placed just under the halfway mark.

The athlete begins the lift from the chosen pin placement, then lowers the bar under control back to the pins before pressing again. The form should be the same as that of the full-range press, so the athlete must pay close attention to avoid compensatory patterns or partial repetition–specific habits.

Dumbbell Press

Using dumbbells in the overhead press forces both arms to work equally in the movement. In this way, imbalances in strength and stability can be addressed. While it may not be possible to press as much weight overhead with dumbbells as it is with a barbell, dumbbells are more unstable than barbells, therefore challenging shoulder stability and increasing deltoid activation, even at a lower weight (Saeterbakken and Fimland 2013).

It is important to note that in a barbell overhead press the hands are fixed in place, whereas in a dumbbell press the arms are free to move in any way they please. Therefore, using dumbbells will not replicate the path of the barbell. This may be useful as an alternative exercise to reduce stress on the shoulders and to minimize the effects of repetitive stress in the barbell overhead press.

Push Press

The push press (see page 43 for more detail) is an excellent way to get a heavier weight overhead than an athlete can press with no leg drive. This movement can also help a longer-armed lifter power past sticking points and potentially lock a weight out more quickly than they would in a strict press. Adding speed to the press can reduce the opportunity for fatigue to set in in the longer bar path inherent in the longer-armed press. The push press can also be useful to strengthen the torso musculature (Bishop, Chavda, and Turner 2018), making it a useful exercise for lifters with long torsos as well.

Overhead Press: Big All Over

Having a large body is definitely an advantage in the overhead press as far as how much weight the lifter can manage. However, there may be some flexibility challenges with larger arms and shoulders. While having a big-all-over body type doesn't necessarily mean that issues with mobility are a given, it's not uncommon to have trouble getting the arms in the right position in an overhead press. And, of course, shoulder mobility issues can exist for lifters of any body type.

The next examples provide optimal overhead press variations for long arms or for lifters with flexibility and mobility limitations. The dumbbell press and landmine press are excellent movements for this category of lifter. In addition, these athletes may find the following movements useful.

Trap Bar Pin Press

The trap bar pin press has a number of benefits for the larger lifter. The structure of the apparatus does not force the lifter into an internally rotated grip—instead, the trap bar allows for a neutral grip, which many big-all-over lifters or those with mobility issues find more comfortable. In addition, setting the bar on pins for each lift allows the bar to remain in a reasonable range of motion for that particular lifter's abilities. Athletes can adjust the pins lower if they wish to practice the push press in this lift.

Log Press

Strongman athletes are among the largest in the world (Kraemer et al. 2020), and the strongman's log may be an ideal apparatus for big-all-over body types. The log provides a neutral grip, like the trap bar, which many lifters with shoulder mobility issues or injuries may find useful. It also sits farther from the touchpoint on the body because of its bulk, therefore requiring a shorter range of motion than a typical barbell. Although the clean and press is generally standard for a log lift in the sport of strongman, many logs are built so they can be racked on a squat cage, so it's possible to simply press the bar from the rack position rather than cleaning it first.

For pressers who tend to lean backward, the log press requires more of a backward lean—head tilted backward, eyes up, lats flared, upper arms as parallel to the floor as possible so that the elbows point in front of the lifter (figure 8.6a). From there, the lifter can strict-press or push-press the log to get it overhead in the fashion desired. The final position is similar to the barbell overhead press—arms should be locked out, and the head should be pushed through the arms so the upper arms are about even with the ears (figure 8.6b).

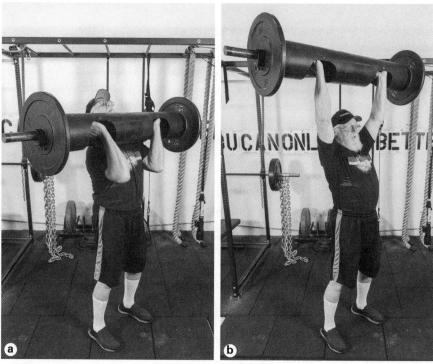

FIGURE 8.6   Log press: start position (a), and finish (b).

Overhead Press: Short Arms

Short-armed lifters, much like with the bench press, may benefit from movements that make the press less efficient. Pausing the press for a few seconds at the chest, or at the pins in a pin press, can be a useful way to reduce efficiency of the press and help break through strength plateaus for the short-armed lifter. Pressing against pins can also be a great way to improve explosive overhead strength for the short-armed lifter and help work through sticking points.

Best Variation: Pressing Against Pins

In this exercise, an empty bar can be used. The lifter sets the safety bars or pins at or slightly above the weakest point of their press (or at any height desired, depending on the position the athlete would like to train). When the barbell reaches the pins or safety bars, the lifter continues to press "through" the blockade as hard as they can, for anywhere from 5 to 30 seconds (figure 8.7). Because this is an absolute maximal effort, the lifter does not need to repeat the movement at that angle on that training day. If another repetition is desired, the lifter should rest accordingly.

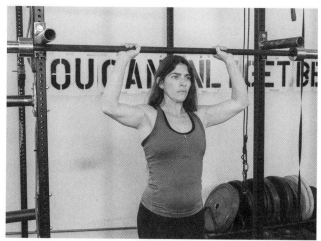

FIGURE 8.7   Pressing against pins.

Ideal Supplementary Lifts to Aid the Overhead Press

Considering the demand of the overhead press—the need for vertical pressing strength and development of the deltoids group and triceps while maintaining a neutral (not extended) spine—the following exercises can be very useful in supplementing the overhead press movement:

- Chinese plank
- Ab wheel rollout
- Single-arm dumbbell snatch
- Dumbbell lateral raise
- French press

Accessory movements can drastically improve the performance of any lift. In the overhead press, strong triceps and a strong, stable base of support are of particular importance. We discuss the details of these assistance exercises in chapter 12.

Chapter 9

The Chin-Up

In practice, many people consider the bench press to be the go-to measure of upper body strength, but looking at the particulars and requirements of the bench press, you can see it's not as important as other lifts. Where pressing exercises are concerned, the overhead press provides more functionality and promotes better joint health. There are also fewer ways to cheat the range of motion or technique in the overhead press, which ends up making it a more difficult lift that you can either perform strongly or not. With that said, as far as premier determinants of upper body strength, we believe there's very little that can compare to the chin-up pattern.

The chin-up pattern is a no-cheating exercise that, regardless of technique, requires a great deal of upper body strength to perform unassisted. It's a testament to the strength of the posterior chain, particularly the muscles of the upper and middle back. Of course, because of the vertical pulling pattern, the biceps musculature also plays a major role in the successful completion of a strong chin-up.

Of note, the chin-up and the pull-up are often mistaken for one another, but you can distinguish them by the hand position. Chin-ups involve a supinated (palms facing the body) position using an underhand grip (figure 9.1a). Pull-ups are performed with a prone (palms away from the body) position, using an overhand grip (figure 9.1b). In the case of pull-ups, the hand width chosen is typically slightly wider than that of a chin-up because of the comfort level each places on the wrists and elbows. Although we're highlighting the chin-up here since it's the more popularly and commonly seen of the two variations, most of the cues listed apply to pull-ups also.

In typical form, the chin-up requires the arms to be completely extended for the start position and the face to clear the bar to the fullest possible elbow flexion for the finish position. Recruitment of upper back and lat musculature depends greatly on how well a lifter can "set the shoulders," or depress and retract the shoulder blades as the lift is in progress. Of course, some considerations need to be made depending on the body type in question.

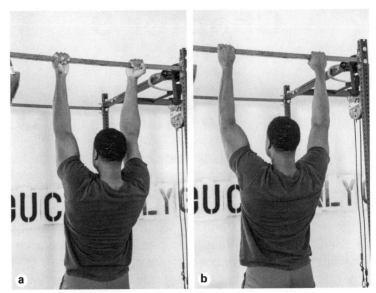

FIGURE 9.1   Chin-up hand position *(a)*, and pull-up hand position *(b)*.

The Perfect Chin-Up Body Type

Moving a shorter distance from point A to point B will make for a stronger chin-up. This prerequisite doesn't mean cutting available range of motion but rather having the proportions conducive to a short distance traveled. The limbs in motion are the arms, and for that reason, shorter arms as a whole will allow for a shorter time under tension and a stronger chin-up. Moreover, the chin-up is a body-weight exercise in its purest form and therefore a demonstration of relative strength over absolute strength. In chapter 2, you learned that smaller, lighter, trained individuals have the capacity to possess more relative strength, whereas heavier, larger lifters have the capacity to possess more absolute strength. Holding true to this concept of absolute versus relative strength, a lighter individual will be better fit for the chin-up. But let's take things one step further.

The chin-up also requires a fair amount of body control. Since the body is suspended off the ground as it hangs from the chin-up bar, it's quite easy for the body to begin swinging uncontrollably as reps progress. A taller, longer person can expend plenty of excess energy simply trying to quiet the unwanted movement to focus on the strict up-and-down pattern a chin-up asks for. For that reason, a lifter with a shorter overall body can also excel at chin-ups. In sum, an individual who's shorter in height, with short extremities relative to their body and a low overall body weight (for more relative strength), would be the ideal body type for chin-up performance.

Chin-Ups: Tall; Long Arms

Because of the great range of motion lifters in these categories need to travel, it's important to first take a look at the intent of chin-ups and then consider the necessary biomechanics of the exercise. A lifter with a tall overall height or with long arms will likely experience a tremendous amount of time under tension traveling from the start position to the finish position. This giant range of motion will lead to an earlier point of fatigue (reps wise) and probably plenty of biceps fatigue since the elbow joint goes through great flexion. For most lifters after strength or muscular development, the intent of adding chin-ups or pull-ups to a program is to train the back musculature as the primary group. Doing so successfully is contingent on using proper technique (mentioned earlier and also in chapter 3).

If we can agree that the latissimus muscles are the prime movers in a chin-up and ultimately the area of focus, then it's worth considering where these muscles attach. Their insertion point is on the intertubercular groove of the humerus—up high on the upper arm (figure 9.2). Anatomically speaking, this insertion point doesn't change, and where that groove is located from person to person is very consistent, regardless of the length of the humerus. In other words, the insertion point of the latissimus isn't completely to scale with the length of the upper arm. Long extremities still result in a fairly similar point of insertion. Even a difference of a few millimeters or even a centimeter or two doesn't account for a difference of 12 or 15 inches (30-38 cm) in wingspan when comparing individuals with long arms against those with shorter arms. This all builds to the question: At what arm angle does the point of greatest lat contraction occur when a lifter has longer arms?

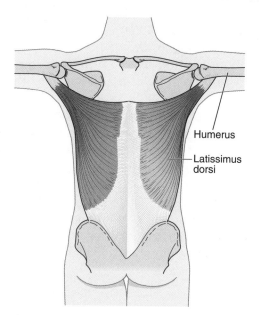

Humerus

Latissimus dorsi

FIGURE 9.2   Latissimus muscles attached to the humerus bone.

On a longer arm, there will probably be more space between the lat attachment and the elbow, compared with a shorter arm. This means that during a chin-up motion for someone with long arms, the lat may shorten to full contraction while the elbow is still farther away from the torso—even by a couple of inches.

Forcing a greater range of motion than your lats are responsible for will only encourage other muscles like the upper traps and biceps to employ themselves even more to help out. This isn't a bad thing in and of itself—these muscles are part of the movement—but the more they are involved, the more a lifter will limit their lat development. This indicates that a longer-armed lifter would benefit most from stopping a few vital inches shy of full range of motion, using a feeling of full contraction as the new landmark,

rather than physical structures like the torso contacting the bar as the end point. Stepping away from such cues can mean only the mouth may clear the bar rather than the entire head and neck. And there's an additional reason why this is so important: shoulder glide.

In an ideal setting, the head of the humerus is in a position of joint centration in the glenoid fossa—that's the ball-and-socket joint known as the shoulder. But especially through deep ranges of shoulder extension, that centration can be lost, and the humeral head can begin sliding forward so the lifter is bearing load in an unfavorable position for such a vulnerable joint (figure 9.3). This humeral position is often seen when people do dips off the edge of a bench (figure 9.4a).

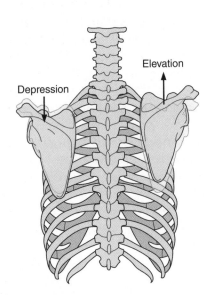

FIGURE 9.3   Shoulder blades in elevated and depressed placement.

Where possible, shoulder glide should be avoided, and the shoulder extension required in a chin-up isn't exempt from this consideration (figure 9.4b). Once the lats reach full contraction, the upper traps' involvement will begin elevating the shoulder blade (this is their function), pulling the shoulder out of its ideal depressed position to finish the lift. Reaching for more range of motion will cause the shoulder to finish out of position, which is not helpful to the lift or the body. For a lifter with shorter arms, this is much less of an issue than for a lifter with longer arms and a greater range of motion to travel. This is why using landmarks like "sternum to bar" is not reliable.

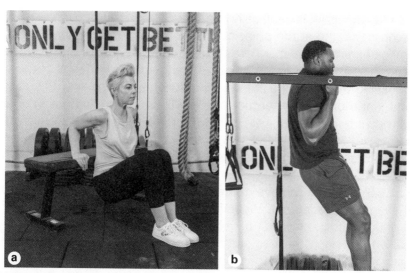

FIGURE 9.4 Shoulder glide in finish position of bench dip (a), and shoulder glide in finish position of chin-up (b).

Best Variation: Flexed Arm Hang

We've chosen an isometric exercise as the primary variation for chin-ups for a couple of reasons. First, the amount of time spent under tension in full lat contraction is unmatched when compared with traditional isotonic reps. Normal chin-ups see this part of the range of motion for only an instant. Also, this variation prevents the biceps from entering the picture to a degree greater than ideal, and it also allows a lifter to customize the starting position.

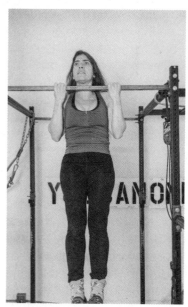

To perform a flexed arm hang, the lifter positions themselves under a bar, in closer-than-normal proximity to the bar itself (this is typically accomplished by standing on a step or box). Next, the lifter uses the step or box to jump up to the top position of the chin-up, where the goal is to hold the position in the fully contracted state for the desired amount of time (figure 9.5). It's easy to allow the shoulders to begin moving out of this position (elevated and with protracted scapulae), so the emphasis must be on maintaining a proud chest and long neck.

FIGURE 9.5 Flexed arm hang finish position.

One reason this lift is especially important for long-armed lifters is that the isometric is created at the point of max contraction. Compare that with an isometric deadlift or squat, where the isometric is typically performed at the start of the concentric rep, completely changing the demands of the movement. Having the isometric at max contraction is a good way to strengthen the end range of the concentric, which will undoubtedly be a struggle for long-armed lifters in the chin-up pattern, and it also creates the extra mobility needed to get the most out of that lifter's active range of motion. Stopping shy of the torso during chin-ups may indeed be in order, but this also means the muscles aren't competing against one another in strength balance, and the joint can properly achieve ranges of motion that it should be able reach. If, for example, the lats are weak in comparison with the tightness of the chest or upper traps, it won't take as much pulling space for shoulder glide to take effect, since the lats can't contract strongly enough to overcome the early forward migration of the upper arm. Although this migration may be inevitable, it may very well occur later than we think.

Doing isometrics with the goal of 30- to 45-second holds is a smart place to begin and should lead to great improvements in pulling strength, muscular endurance, technique, and back hypertrophy.

Rack Chin-Up

As mentioned, unwanted swinging can be an issue in chin-ups and is often amplified when a greater range of motion is in the mix. For that reason, gently banking the feet on an object, like a step or box, can be a game changer to establish control without providing too much assistance.

The idea with the rack chin-up is for the legs to take some of the loading off the body, which can result in a stricter chin-up with more isolation toward the upper and middle back. As an aside, this is a great option for lifters who are most concerned with adding muscle size to their backs. This can also help lifters in this category focus on a brief pause, or isometric hold, at the top of each repetition.

To properly perform rack chin-ups, a lifter has a couple of options. First, they can set up with a bench or step at a standard chin-up bar and use that as their surface to place the feet on (figure 9.6a). As long as the surface is high enough to allow the legs to bend to nearly a 90-degree angle when the arms are fully extended, this is allowable. In the case of rack chin-ups, the most standard setup would be for the step (and the feet) to be positioned ever so slightly behind the bar (and body). Pressing gently with the legs as the pull is made toward the top position adds just the amount of assistance and control necessary to complete the lift with maximum isolation (figure 9.6b).

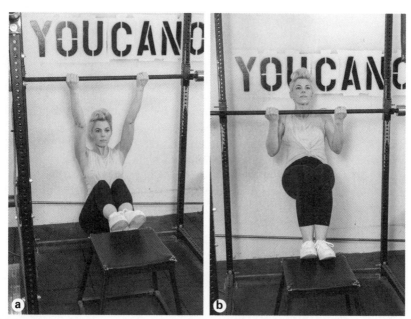

FIGURE 9.6 Rack chin-up: start position *(a)*, and finish *(b)*.

Chin-Ups: Big All Over

In the case of lifters who are heavier and larger, the issue might not be the frustration of a given technical element of the lift—it could be the frustration of overall size and heavy weight making it difficult to complete reps. For big, heavy lifters, their relative strength will be exploited with this exercise, and despite great performances in other movements like the squat and deadlift, chin-up or pull-up performance often suffers. There's no other explanation to be made, other than the sad truth that those are the breaks when you carry a whole lot of mass.

With this in mind, it would be ambitious to give a list of advanced chin-up variations so lifters of this demographic can take things to the next level. The reality is, technique would likely break down in a hurry. As a back-dominant exercise, the chin-up should be a movement a lifter can perform for reps to tap into the necessary muscular endurance of their postural muscles. It's up to the lifter to choose the right exercises to make that possible.

Best Variation: Eccentric Chin-Up

Adding time to an eccentric rep of any exercise will strengthen a lifter's ability on both halves of a lift. Exhausting muscle fibers in the concentric portion of an exercise still leaves a large amount of a lifter's capacity untapped. To illustrate: If a lifter said their max-effort bench press was 315 pounds (140 kg) for one rep, that would lead you, the listener, to naturally conclude that

Kyphosis

It is worth a brief segue to discuss a spinal dysfunction known as kyphosis. We touch on mobility issues in chapter 2, when examining the spine closely. Kyphosis affects the thoracic spine, which is the upper and middle back (figure 9.7*a*), and causes a rounded posture (figure 9.7*b*). Most people think it affects only the spine, but this change in spinal shape has an impact on the rest of the back and the rib cage as well. The position of the scapulae on a thoracic spine and rib cage under kyphosis will definitely shift, pushing them higher and outward into a more dysfunctional winged position. Along with this change, the front side of the body often becomes chronically short and tight because of the closed rib cage position and protracted shoulders. This can contribute to shoulder pain, and more importantly, it can contraindicate chin-ups.

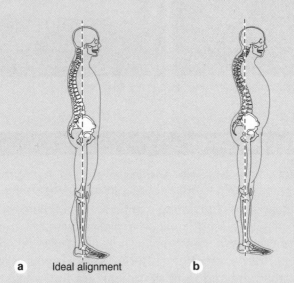

a   Ideal alignment   b

Figure 9.7   Example of ideally aligned spine *(a)*, and kyphosis-lordosis spine *(b)*.

When it comes to back exercises, people think any choice is a good one where development, shoulder health, and postural correction are concerned. And the logic is tempting: Strengthen the upper back, open up the front side, and create balance. In good intention, people will double up on their pulling movements, which can include chin-ups, reasoning they are premier strengthening exercises that also have a huge positive impact on posture and are better for shoulder health.

When someone's spine is chronically flexed to the point of kyphosis, however, standard body-weight chin-ups might not be the best choice. With the winged scapular position typical of a hunched posture, a person will have an incomplete range of flexion for the arm at the shoulder joint. Reaching overhead for any movement will result in compensation, usually at the lower back (figure 9.8*a*). Forcing the arms into a dead hang position under a pull-up

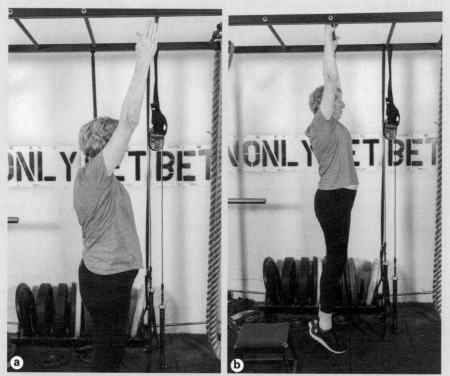

Figure 9.8   Kyphotic spine and incomplete shoulder flexion *(a)*, and Kyphotic spine hanging under bar with full shoulder flexion *(b)*.

bar may seem like a good way to build range of motion, but in reality, it's a big compromise to shoulder health for an immobile lifter (figure 9.8*b*). If a lifter can't get to that position naturally, then fixing the hands to a bar to hang into that position isn't a true solution.

This issue can be resolved by modifying the rack chin-up. Changing the platform for the rack chin-up from behind the body to in front allows a lifter to place their entire body on a slight backward lean, which can better accommodate insufficient shoulder mobility and still train an overhead pull pattern using body weight as resistance. Assuming a pike or V-sit position with the legs straight out in front of the body (heels on the platform or box) allows for a more comfortable torso angle while still providing mild assistance from the legs. Alternatively, moving the box a few inches closer to the body and starting with bent legs is another option for those who find it more comfortable to do so. Above all things, a kyphotic spine may require attention from an appropriate practitioner, depending on the severity of the kyphosis. Since the overwhelming majority of weight training exercises require the ability to keep a tall spine and the shoulders held back, it can present unwanted risk if this position can't be achieved, or the position of thoracic flexion can't be overcome. If this applies to your client, it's best to take the responsible route and get clearance for training by a sports therapist or physical therapist.

giving that lifter 320 or 325 pounds (145 or 147 kg) would leave them unable to press the weight away from the chest. However, if that lifter with the same max effort of 315 was asked to take that 325-pound bar and lower it slowly to the chest, without pressing it up afterward, the possibility of doing that successfully would be very high (almost certain).

This goes to show that everyone possesses more eccentric strength (strength on the lowering phase of a movement) than they do concentric strength. Because of this strength bias, working hard to exhaust and train those portions of a given lift can only improve a lifter's total strength in a movement—and expose that lifter to plenty of time under tension while at it. Eccentric chin-ups pull no punches when it comes to the training effect they deliver, and specific to big and heavy lifters, they certainly require no additional loading beyond body weight. The aim of the lift is to never sacrifice full range of motion and also to do zero work during the concentric phase of the movement.

After setting up a box or step under the chin-up bar, slightly behind, to the side of, or in front of the body, a lifter stands on top of it so the distance between the head and the bar is fairly close. Next, the lifter jumps up to the top position with the hands in chin-up grip. Ideally, the shoulders will be set down and back to mimic the finish position of any vertical pulling pattern. After this, the lifter attempts to "brake" the free descent, lowering slowly toward the floor until the arms are in a fully extended position and the body is in a true dead hang. This means that on the way down, the lifter will ignore the box or step that was used to boost the concentric phase. The lifter then steps up to the box and repeats. Focusing on sets of three to six reps is ideal, since it will not take much more than this to lose eccentric control. On that note, the goal should be for a lifter's descent to be between 5 and 10 seconds per rep. This is usually easier said than done.

To make this movement more challenging, a lifter can add eccentric isometrics by pausing at various segments throughout the descent. Pausing for 3 to 5 seconds at the quarter point, halfway point, and three-quarter point of the eccentric rep can add even more time under tension and exhaust the muscle fibers.

Neutral-Grip Chin-Up and Ring Chin-Up

Broad shoulders and substantial arm size and mass often go hand in hand with some form of mobility restriction, and this isn't limited to mobility of the shoulder or hip joints. The elbow and wrist joints may not be able to fully supinate, especially when being asked to tether the hands to a bar in a fixed position. Similar to a chin-up with a kyphotic spine, what may appear to be a sufficient level of flexibility when hanging under the bar may not amount to the same amount of achievable range of motion when free-handed (without using a landmark or gravitational forces to help achieve said position).

If a lifter has access to a neutral grip for chin-ups, this is a smart modification for a more comfortable pulling position for big lifters (figure 9.9a-b). There is some concern whether there's a significant change in muscle activation depending on hand grip, but the differences in back and lat activity between variations are too small to be noteworthy (Dickie et al. 2017). Alternatively, using a grip that changes through the force curve (from neutral to supine) by way of gymnastics rings is a recommended option to service the natural comfortable position for the chin-up grip. Starting in a neutral grip and finishing with a palms-in grip can feel much better than remaining in one of the two for the entire duration of the movement, and using this grip variety comes with no muscular disadvantage in performing the lift (Youdas et al. 2010).

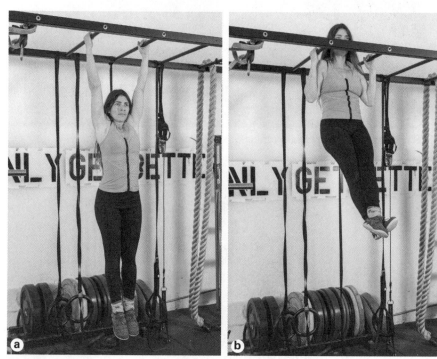

FIGURE 9.9 Neutral-grip chin-up: start position (a), and finish (b).

If your gym setup doesn't include gymnastics rings (figure 9.10a-b), an investment in portable rotating grips to tie around a fixed bar is a smart and inexpensive alternative. Many cable machines use nylon-based hand grips that can be borrowed for the same purposes, as long as the straps are long enough (figure 9.11).

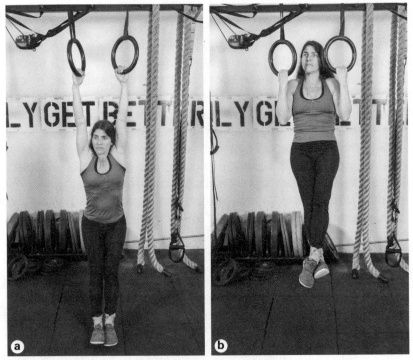

FIGURE 9.10   Gymnastics ring chin-up: start position *(a)*, and finish *(b)*.

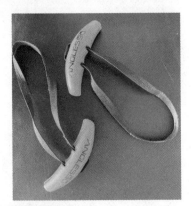

FIGURE 9.11   Rotating grips.

Band-Assisted Chin-Up or Pull-Up

As mentioned, many big lifters may be strong in other movements but struggle to move their body weight. Using a band not only enables a lifter to perform more repetitions of the exercise but also makes a key adjustment to the resistance profile. Tying a band around the chin-up bar and stretching it under the foot acts as a sling to assist the movement (figure 9.12a-b). Since the band is the most stretched when the lifter is nearest the floor, the beginning phases of the pattern will receive the most help from the band, whereas the ending phases will receive the least. We believe this is the perfect resistance profile for a heavy lifter to take advantage of.

When in a dead hang, lifters who struggle with chin-ups and pull-ups typically tend to jerk or kip their way into creating inertia to start the movement, but this is not a good habit to adopt. Remember, the hands are stuck in one place, meaning the joint that takes the brunt of these forces is the shoulder. There's no other load-bearing joint that a similar initiation of loaded movement would be considered safe for, and there's also no joint less stable than the shoulder. These facts are not a good combination. For that reason, having a bit of extra help until proper form can be achieved without a band is in proper order.

Beyond that, on the topic of back isolation, using a band to take some of the weight away from chin-ups can be beneficial for bodybuilding purposes. If the addition of assistance to the movement can change a set of 6 or 7 reps into a set of 10 or 12 reps (or a greater number of total sets before complete exhaustion), with better form to boot, it's worth looking into. This means more total volume and a greater chance to develop the upper and middle back.

Of course, this is all to be taken with a grain of salt. Keep in mind that bands come in varying widths and thicknesses. It wouldn't make sense to use a band far too thick for band-assisted chin-ups; that would be the equivalent of a bench press spotter who takes it upon themselves to carry half the lifter's weight on each rep. Find the thickness that enables comple-

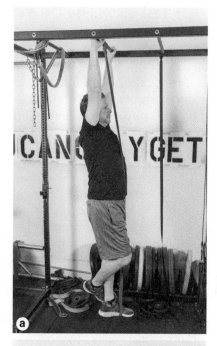
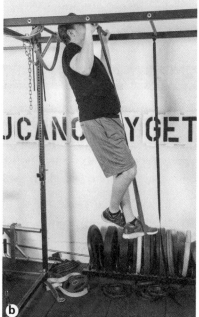

FIGURE 9.12 Band-assisted pull-up: start position *(a)*, and finish *(b)*.

tion of the target number of reps in question while maintaining good form. Those reps should mostly rely on the strength of the body, not the strength of the band.

For best results, use a loop band. The band is hung around the chin-up bar (or the support structure that houses the neutral-grip chin-up bar, depending on the apparatus' setup) and looped through itself for a proper and secure anchor point. Lifters typically stretch the band under either the bent knee or the foot (figure 9.12a); if possible, we recommend the foot, since this means more assistance and a deeper stretch to the band, and it also lets the body remain straighter under the bar without being forced into a bent-knee position. With the bands under one foot, the option to cross the legs still exists (figure 9.12b).

The Hard Truth

Bigger lifters need to keep in mind that all of these coaching cues may help, but one real issue at play is their size. If improving pull-up or chin-up performance is a true goal of practicing the exercise, it shouldn't be completely off the table to consider a reduction of mass or body weight to help the cause. Especially if body fat levels are higher, this can be beneficial for any lifter looking to improve pull-up or chin-up performance. But even in the case of lean individuals, this is one of the instances where more muscle and more size aren't necessarily the greatest thing. This may be a tough pill to swallow, but it needed to be written and read. It likely won't be advice you'll find in another book focused on strength training.

Chin-Ups: Short; Short Arms

The overwhelming issue with lifters who have a small range of motion when performing chin-ups and pull-ups is the fact they usually feel their backs can handle more than what their arms can offer in each rep. It's difficult to find ways to create more range of motion or pulling space in a chin-up; the arms can only reach so far. With that said, it's worth remembering two facts:

1. The lats are internal rotators of the upper arm.
2. A greater stretch can happen unilaterally.

For those reasons, the following exercises are great choices for strength and hypertrophy.

Best Variation: Sternum Chin-Up or Pull-Up

Especially with a neutral grip, this chin-up variation forces plenty of comfortable added range of motion. Since the lats internally rotate the humerus, coupling the overhead pulling pattern with a horizontal pull while squeezing the hands toward each other can make for an intense lat contraction and double as a great core strength developer (figure 9.13). Since the body finishes much more horizontal to the floor compared with a typical chin-up, this exercise places a demand on more muscles than just those of the upper and middle back.

Like the name suggests, the lifter assumes a typical hanging start position on the chin-up bar and pulls toward the top while aiming for the sternum (midchest) to make it closest to the bar—not the chin or face. The lifter must add a bit of arch to the upper back and lean backward with the body to achieve this. For a lifter with a short overall body height (and typically not the heaviest body weight overall), this finishing position is definitely achievable if there's a good base of strength and conditioning. One added coaching cue worth mentioning is to make an extra effort to contract the glutes. This will counter any back stress

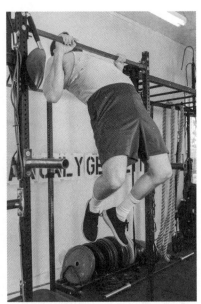

FIGURE 9.13 Sternum pull-up.

the aggressive arch could potentiate, and it will also help brace the entire posterior chain for better levering and greater control on the way up and down, with less unwanted swinging.

This movement, because of its extreme range of motion, will take more energy per rep and can't be performed for the same rep range as normal chin-ups. For that reason, lowering reps by around 30 percent is a good directive to follow.

Band-Assisted Single-Arm Chin-Up

Doing a one-armed chin-up has always been a calisthenic feat of strength attainable by few. Admittedly, these are fairly difficult for even the best of lifters, but modifying things by adding a band allows a lifter to focus on one key element: the amount of additional stretch the lat can go through when one arm gets to reach higher than the other.

This is the reason a one-handed slam dunk in basketball is easier for an athlete to attain than a two-handed slam dunk. The body has the opportunity to reach farther when the movement isn't bilateral. This can be a saving grace for lat training and unilateral strength using the length–tension relationship.

Performing these chin-ups requires the same initial setup of attaching a loop band to the chin-up bar. This time we recommend securing the band around both feet instead of just one. Using a very narrow, supinated grip, the lifter lowers the body to a full hang and then removes one hand (figure 9.14a). It's acceptable—and recommended—to place the free hand on the forearm of the working side. Doing so will steady the body from too much swaying or rocking to keep the movement linear in nature without much accessory movement. The next step is to simply pull through a full chin-up

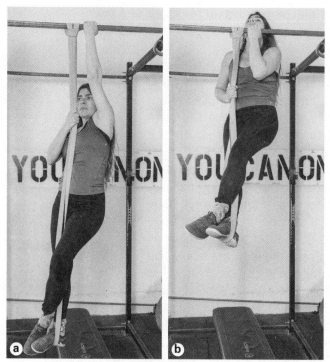

FIGURE 9.14   Single-arm banded chin-up: start position *(a)*, and finish *(b)*.

range of motion (figure 9.14*b*). The body will likely twist toward the side of the working arm, and that's acceptable as long as it's not excessive.

For this exercise, a thicker band is ideal, since one arm is bearing more load than normal, even with assistance. Making up for a small range of motion by using higher reps per arm is also recommended, so focusing on sets of eight or more reps can go a long way in developing the back and biceps.

Weighted Chin-Up

We made it clear that the ideal body type to perform chin-ups well is the shorter demographic, or at the very least the demographic with shorter arms. For that reason it should be taken advantage of if the skills are present. One would be hard pressed to find many people who are well over 200 pounds (90 kg) who are also excellent at pull-ups and chin-ups. Those people may be strong enough to crack out a few reps of weighted chin-ups, but it's likely they're not absolutely necessary to help improve strength. A 260-pound (120 kg) body making its way over the bar is more than enough.

However, when levers are shorter, range of motion is smaller, and body mass is lower, this often creates the stage for more progression of the lift in its basic form, by the numbers. Adding a weight belt or weighted vest and performing chin-ups or pull-ups using external loading can prove useful to unlock more strength gains (figure 9.15*a-b*). This can also be achieved using band resistance (figure 9.16*a-b*) to change the resistance profile (which would make the lift most difficult at the top of the concentric portion).

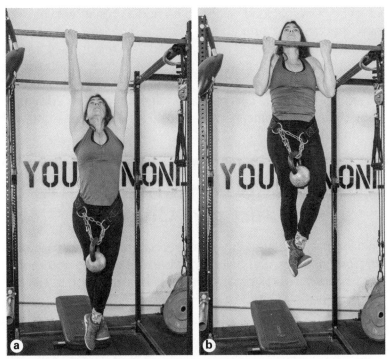

FIGURE 9.15   Weight belt chin-up: start position *(a)*, and finish *(b)*.

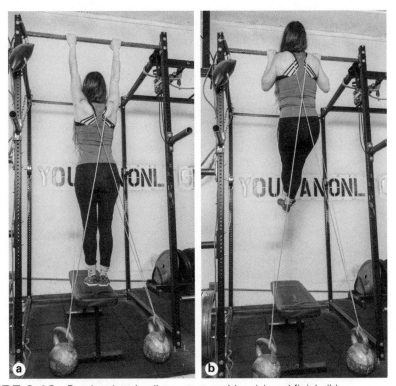

FIGURE 9.16   Band-resisted pull-up: start position *(a)*, and finish *(b)*.

In each case, external load needs to be added conservatively. Too many lifters think that simply being able to get the face over the bar is the only thing required for chin-ups and pull-ups, and as a result, they add plenty of external load to their pull-ups or chin-ups. But if form and technique can't be respected by following the coaching cues listed in chapter 3, then nothing should be added until they can be. An addition of a mere 20 extra pounds (10 kg) should make a significant difference if lifting honestly and with a feel for technique.

Ideal Supplementary Lifts to Aid the Chin-Up

Vertical pulling patterns are fairly simple in overall demand and execution, and aside from chin-ups and pull-ups themselves, some common lifts can be of aid to improve overall back strength and arm flexion strength:

- Biceps curl variations
- Lat pull-down
- Row variations
- Hanging leg raise

It's of supreme importance to a lifter's mobility, upper body strength, lifting prowess, and even physique to become proficient at vertical pulls (in this case, the chin-up or pull-up patterns). In and of itself, the movement is fairly black and white; you can either complete the rep or you can't—quite similar to the deadlift. With that said, applying the principles specific to the body type in question can be a very effective route toward letting a lifter nail their first pull-up or break through a plateau that adds a few extra reps to their total. Either way, it's an upper body movement that certainly shouldn't be neglected, regardless of the training goal.

Chapter 10

The Row Pattern

This chapter shares a few similarities with chapter 9, mainly because the chin-up and row are both back-dominant, upper body pulling patterns. With that said, there are more particulars about rows that lifters would be prudent to recognize.

Row patterns, first and foremost, have slightly more universal application because fewer populations will lack the mobility to pull horizontally relative to the torso compared with vertically. In other words, a row pattern is less contingent on a healthy full range of circumduction (especially flexion) at the shoulder joint, compared with a chin-up or pull-up. With that in mind, every AC joint classification (discussed in prior chapters) would be able to find multiple rowing variations that cause no pain to the lifter.

Since there are so many row variations, it's sensible to categorize them. First, it's worthwhile to consider the most popular versions of the row pattern and work in reverse, so to speak, to determine what body types best fit the pattern in question. The rowing movements we've seen most in our experience can be narrowed down to three lifts: seated cable rows, bent-over rows, and single-arm dumbbell rows. These patterns are often erroneously performed, making it good for a refresher on technique.

Seated Cable Row

This pattern uses a cable pulley for a very consistent line of force and starting and finishing points with the weights. This can be a benefit for lifters with prior injuries to the spine or lumbar musculature, where irregularities in the bar's path can risk spine safety and briefly create greater stress forces due to a change in force angle. From machine to machine, the structure of the modality may differ; some have higher foot platforms, some have lower. For some machines, the pulley with the cable and attachment is placed exactly in line with the feet, and for others, the pulley is recessed past the feet for the ability to reach farther forward without the stacked plates crashing down (figure 10.1a-b).

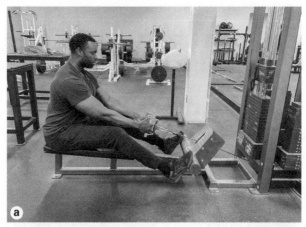

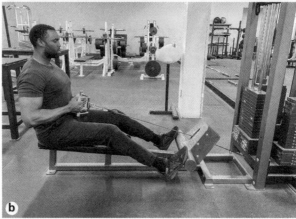

FIGURE 10.1 Seated row with V-grip: start position *(a)*, and finish *(b)*.

For these reasons, as a whole, cable rows can be of great service to lifters who have longer legs, longer arms, and shorter torsos. This isn't to say other body types can't benefit from this variation of the movement. It simply means the constraints of the seated row may be most easily overcome by these body types. A short-legged lifter with a longer torso may be confined by the amount of pulling distance they can create, since the starting point does not allow for much space to stretch forward for the beginning of each rep. Consequentially, in the attempt to get as far away from the pulley as possible, the lifter might straighten the legs to slide the buttocks farther back on the bench. The problem with this modification is that completely straightening the legs can make it much more difficult (and isolated to the most flexible lifters) to avoid flexion in the lumbar spine at any given point of the pattern. Ideally the spine's degree of flexion or extension should barely change despite the change of angle at the hip joint. Even though the force angle on the flexed spine is different from those imposed by a deadlift or squat, it's still an unwanted and less safe position compared with a neutral or slightly extended spine and must be guarded against—especially when lifting heavier loads.

A Guide to Rowing Handles, Hand Placement, and Shoulders

Longer-armed lifters need to take note of shoulder glide and pulling distance, mentioned in the previous chapter on chin-ups. Some of the issue of shoulder glide will depend on the grip and handles used by the lifter (more on that later), but for the most part, the distance a long-armed lifter needs to pull in order to make the handle contact the torso will exceed their shoulders' range of extension. As a result, the lifter could lose their ideal pulling posture, making for a finish position that has the shoulder rolled forward and the chest sunken—instead of the shoulder being in proper joint centration in its socket (figure 10.2).

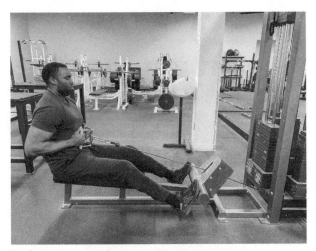

FIGURE 10.2 Seated row with poor posture.

To keep this from happening, a safe directive would be to stop, as for chin-ups, at the point of max contraction of the upper back muscles. The rhomboids, middle and lower traps, rear deltoids, and scapular muscles like the teres major, supraspinatus, and infraspinatus are all target muscles for the row pattern. Since there is less emphasis on the abdominals and overall body control than for a chin-up pattern, it's fair to conclude that the row is far more focused on training and isolating the upper back musculature rather than simply making the lifter more proficient at the athletic pattern. Knowing this, freezing the rep at the point where the working muscles can't get any shorter, which will likely be when the elbows just barely pass beyond the torso on the concentric phase of the lift, will likely translate to the handle *not* being in contact with the torso at the finish point of the rep. Keep in mind that this is fine for a lifter with the proportions we're discussing.

A Closer Look at the Popular V-Grip

The issue of shoulder glide can be amplified according to how medially the handles place the hands relative to the torso. The most common handle attachment is the iron V-grip. It has a very narrow, unforgiving grip position that internally rotates the shoulders to a worsening degree depending on the shoulder width of the lifter holding it. This further drives home the point that stopping shy of full range on each rep can help keep the focus on the upper back and away from the shoulder capsule. Also, replacing the V-grip handle with a pull-down bar attachment can be a smart substitution to enable a wider grip that allows the hands to better align with the elbows and shoulders (figure 10.3a-b). Adding an underhand position to this pattern can externally rotate the upper arm, placing the humeral head in a better spot to encourage joint centration through the range.

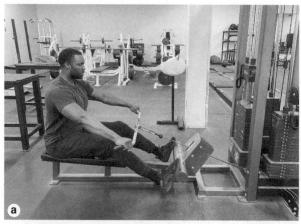

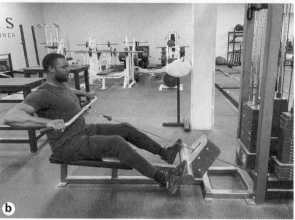

FIGURE 10.3 Wide-grip row with pull-down bar attachment: start position (a), and finish (b).

Barbell Bent-Over Row

This pattern can be performed with a variety of hand positions on the barbell: narrower, wider, with a prone hand position (overhand grip), or with a supine position (underhand grip). What matters across the board is that the elbows remain in line with the hands through the duration of the pull and the straight-line patterning of the bar be preserved. We'll preface the breakdown of this lift by saying it makes a terrific supplement for deadlift strength and performance. Knowing this, a lifter is more likely to excel in this pattern if they've got a solid handle on the deadlift, regardless of the body type. The reason we're mentioning the relationship between bent-over rows and deadlifts is that a bent-over row asks for the entire spine to remain in a neutral or extended position for the duration of the set. There's no time within the set to rest or reset, and as the body fatigues, the spine can lose its flatness and end up flexed. Longer arms to pull means greater time under tension and a greater pulling distance to bring the bar from bottom to top (which is demanding in an unsupported bent-over position).

Note that the geometry of the body may be fairly similar to the starting position of the seated cable row, but the spine will endure a greater magnitude of demand compared with the bent-over row for two reasons: First, the hips are immobilized in a seated row because the buttocks are planted on the seat. Second, the forces of gravity aren't as directly at play in the seated row compared with the bent-over row. Seated rows make the weight move away from the ground by way of a cable attached to pulleys, pulled horizontally. Bent-over rows make the weight move away from the ground by way of the arms lifting the weight directly from ground level to torso level, stabilized by the trunk and posterior chain musculature.

Having said this, a lifter with a longer torso and shorter arms and legs can be best suited for this exercise, so the focus can rightfully be placed on the upper back and less on fighting to achieve the proper spinal position to even begin a lifting set. Likewise, since a bent-over row is performed from a hanging or hovering bar position, a lifter with longer legs can more easily become frustrated by the bar intersecting with the knees when in the transition phases (passing between the eccentric and concentric phases of the lift). Keeping the shins vertical to keep the knees from intersecting with the bar will mean a more horizontal torso position that runs nearly parallel to the floor (figure 10.4a-b). This isn't a bad thing; it simply demands more of a lifter's flexibility, mobility, and lower back strength to maintain technique and produce strong reps. However, a lifter who can't make these changes will end up sitting too tall while rowing, which will shift the emphasis of the movement away from the rhomboids, low traps, rear deltoids, and lats and place it higher up toward the upper traps, since the loaded bar will still be lifted in the same vertical line as before.

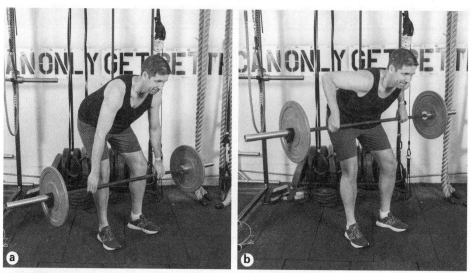

FIGURE 10.4   Bent-over row: start position *(a)*, and finish *(b)*.

Because of the demands of the movement, a lifter could err on the side of caution and safety by wearing a lifting belt when performing the bent-over row pattern. Since there's no true concentric or eccentric component to the lift for the lumbar region nor any break from effort between reps, it could be argued that this pattern demands the use of a lifting belt for support more than a typical deadlift.

Single-Arm Dumbbell Row

Setting up on a bench with a single dumbbell to perform rows often leaves a lifter confused as to what muscles to think about targeting during the lift. Many people think the single-arm dumbbell row functions the same way as seated or bent-over rows. The truth is, from a biomechanical perspective, the hand and arm positions are quite different when the lifts are performed correctly. A proper setup requires one knee to be firmly planted on a bench, with the hand on the same side of the body positioned at the front of the bench. The other foot should be planted squarely on the floor adjacent to the first knee, and the dumbbell should be hanging directly under the shoulder.

For most people, the arm position relative to the torso will be in greater shoulder flexion compared with both seated and bent-over rows. Since the weight is held in a neutral grip and the hand and arm are more medial (or toward the midline of the body), slightly different kinematics are required to perform the pattern, and this will favor different muscles while in action.

Rather than find the best angle to target the upper back muscles the way the row variations do—which would be very frustrating to pinpoint—it's better to let the natural action of the humerus guide the movement in the

Seated Rows and Bent-Over Rows: Dissecting Torso Position and Top Rock

Some movement of the torso is not only allowable but specifically recommended during these rowing patterns. A reasonable amount of upper body movement would not cause any undue risk or be a disservice to the exercise a long as proper spinal position is maintained for the duration of the exercise.

Many will argue that it's imperative to keep the torso rigid during these movements, even if that means using very light weight. Pundits will also insist these row variations require a rigid torso since greater loads can be lifted. Any movement at the hips while rowing—what is sometimes known as *top rock*—would constitute cheating and a conclusion that the weight is too heavy.

On the contrary, incorporating some upper body movement during either of these row patterns can be an effective way of stimulating more back tissue and safely moving more weight. A mobile torso—as compared with a totally stationary one—means the low back isn't forced to maintain an isometric hold through the entire set. In practice, it doesn't make sense that the endurance level of the lower back should determine the effectiveness of the row exercise. Of course, this can be taken overboard—and many people do go too far with it. An overzealous attitude can definitely get in the way of lifting to stimulate the right muscles. Seated rows and barbell bent-over rows are staples in many programs, but they fall prey to excessive momentum, looseness, and the act of just going through the motions in efforts to simply finish the lift. There are several bad ways to compromise form to get the reps up, since it is easy to cheat in row variations.

Mixing bad body geometry with an aggressive top rock makes heavy pulls dangerous. But you would be remiss to think that some form of movement shouldn't be permissible when rowing heavy weight. A 225-pound (100 kg) or heavier bent-over row, for example, would be considered quite an appreciable load for the overwhelming majority of lifters who attempt to move it, let alone with a completely rigid and motionless torso. There's simply a ceiling on how much the arms will be able to pull. As long as the low back stays in a slight arch (the way it should), incorporating a well-timed, tight top rock to start the lift is both beneficial and necessary. It takes practice to learn the timing and to understand just the right amount of top rock that can be used during reps of heavy weight. But to row heavy, it's best to invest the time to learn and teach this method to clients. They may start by doing seated and bent-over rows using the method described earlier with lighter weight.

name of comfort. Shoulder extension from this starting position will move the elbow closer toward the hip, and the dumbbell should follow. Setting the shoulder from this point and truly letting the body not compete against gravity will mean letting the dumbbell follow a slightly arcing or sweeping pattern as the elbow moves. This will make it much easier to avoid shoulder glide and encourage shortening of the back muscles—more specifically, the lats.

Using the single-arm dumbbell row as a lat exercise and less of an upper back exercise may require further explanation. Consider the fibrous path of the muscles of the lats. Their muscle fibers travel neither horizontally nor vertically. They tend to travel in a slanted pattern, and a loaded shoulder extension must correspond with this fibrous path in order to most effectively target the muscle. This logic is what makes the pull-down pattern sister exercise, with its mild torso lean and stiff-arm pull-down, so effective at targeting the same muscle group. In both cases, shoulder extension is met with a corresponding torso angle to keep the lats as the primary mover of the shoulder joint.

Having said all this, the lifter with a longer torso and shorter legs will have a couple of distinct user-friendly advantages when performing single-arm dumbbell rows: First, the ground won't get in the way of full arm extension at the bottom of each rep; the dumbbell will be able to hover over the ground in its transition between eccentric and concentric reps since the arms aren't long enough to reach the floor from a standard bench height. Shorter legs mean the back will be on a slant that travels upward from hip to shoulder, rather than downward, so that the lifter feels as if they're pulling from a decline position. Combining these biomechanics and proportions with a longer torso creates distance between the upper and lower extremities when in the set position for the lift. This is important because a common frustration of the exercise is that the elbow of the working arm collides with the thigh of the grounded leg. A compensation to prevent such a collision involves stepping out of alignment by dropping the grounded leg farther back (thus causing the pelvis to lose its alignment).

Very few setup adjustments help the performance of this exercise, but one noteworthy change is to perform the movement on an adjustable bench rather than a flat one. Adjusting the bench to one level above the flat setting will incline the backrest (and in many cases, slightly incline the seat), which can prove itself to be a much more comfortable setup than remaining flat (figure 10.5a). As a bonus, a hand positioned on a slightly inclined surface makes it easier to keep the rib cage higher, making better use of thoracic spine extension (figure 10.5b). This change can lend to better-quality shoulder blade retraction and more back musculature involvement for more purposeful reps.

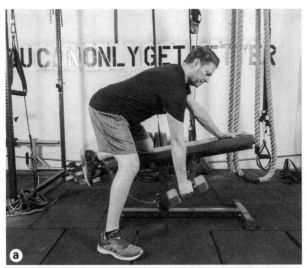

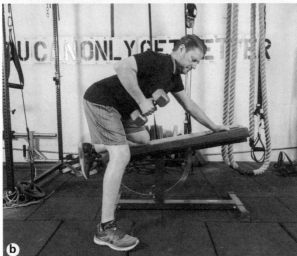

FIGURE 10.5 Single-arm row with adjustable bench: start position *(a)*, and finish *(b)*.

The Rest of Us: Best Row Variations for Other Body Types

Like other lifts, certain variations will cater best to certain body types. Although there are fewer variables and moving parts to row patterns, that same notion applies. A lifter with wider shoulders may not fare the same way as a lifter with longer levers during certain seated row variations. Likewise, a lifter with long arms may be frustrated by their biceps fatiguing earlier than the target back muscles. Using those examples as fair reason, it brings credence to the idea of individuality within the movement.

Rows: Big All Over

When a lifter has plenty of trunk volume from front to back, especially coupled with a whole lot of width, modifications to a classic seated row are in order. Often, the range of motion they can potentially achieve with their scapulae and shoulder joints is blocked by the size of their torso, specifically when the hands are connected to a handle or bar. In the case of the seated row, the V-grip, mentioned earlier, makes the situation worse because of internal rotation at the shoulder (and accompanied shoulder glide). For this reason, it's smart to let each hand move freely, unattached to a central point.

Best Variation: Ring Inverted Row

The inverted row is a body-weight-based movement that's very effective at targeting the upper back musculature and lats, while also being much friendlier to the lower back than other rowing variations (Fenwick et al. 2009). Using rings to perform inverted rows offers many advantages that big lifters can benefit from. First and foremost, individual rings mean no compensation between arms, and the lifter can pull the hands farther than a bar would allow. Whereas the torso would typically touch the bar before the elbows pass the body, the hands now have the chance to finish at the actual point of peak contraction of the upper back musculature (and peak retraction of the shoulder blades), which is likely farther than the confines of the bar or V-grip row variations can allow. If rings aren't available, suspension straps like TRX could provide a substitute.

In addition to this, ring inverted rows allow for much-needed play room for the elbow and wrist positions. Similar to the ring chin-ups mentioned in chapter 9, using rings to row can encourage a lifter to rotate the hands on each pull, which, above all else, can be much more comfortable than remaining neutral, internally rotated, or externally rotated. Of course, gymnastics rings mean the need for greater stability, but that should be welcome since the risk to the shoulder is lowered, given this is a pulling variation and not a pressing variation.

Manipulating the resistance for a gymnastics ring inverted row is a commonly asked question, and big lifters will notice that it doesn't take much to get a great workout using body weight alone. A lifter can choose to perform these inverted rows with the feet flat on the ground and a 90-degree knee bend (figure 10.6a-b) or with the legs straight and only the heels in contact with the floor (which would be more challenging with all else equal). Moreover, the more directly underneath the rings the lifter sets up, the greater the percentage of body weight they will bear. That percentage decreases the more the lifter remains standing. For lifters seeking an additional challenge that body weight alone cannot provide, there are two more options at their disposal.

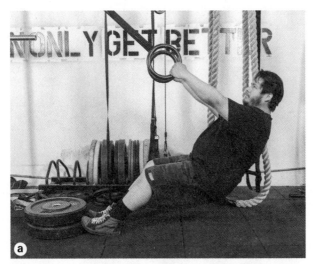

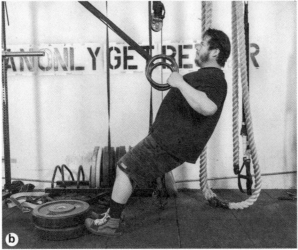

FIGURE 10.6   Bent-knee ring row: start position *(a)*, and finish *(b)*.

Elevate the Heels

Raising the heels above floor level so that the shoulders are in line with (or below) the feet further increases the difficulty level of the exercise because it increases the percentage of body weight lifted. Again, opting between a bent-knee position (figure 10.7a) (with the feet flat on the raised surface) or a stiff-legged position (figure 10.7b) (with only the heels on the raised surface) can create different levels of intensity in this advanced training method.

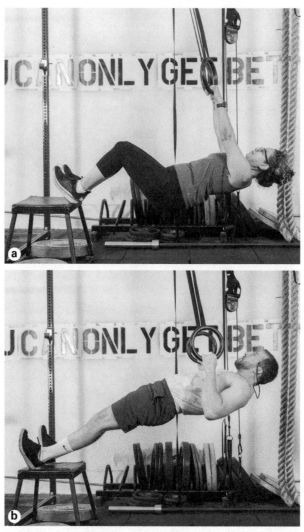

FIGURE 10.7   Heels-elevated ring rows with bent knees *(a)*, and with straight knees *(b)*.

Wear a Weighted Vest

If the lifter wants an even more challenging option to promote muscle and strength
development, adding a weighted vest
(figure 10.8) can be the next course of
action. Of note, however, many weighted
vests—even depending on the size of
the vest—can restrict the free motion of
the upper body, specifically in overhead,
pulling, and pushing motions. This can be
made worse if the body wearing the vest
is also very large or wide. Doing diligence
to select a weighted vest that allows as
much freedom of mobility through the
upper back and shoulder capsule is important to enable proper row technique while
wearing it.

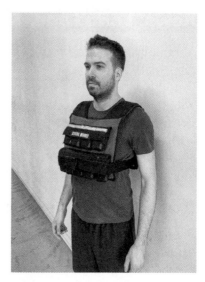

FIGURE 10.8 Weighted vest.

As a reminder, the goal with all these variations does not change to gear-
ing for a 5-rep max. These are still rows, and as such, they deserve to be
trained for higher rep ranges. Focusing on sets of 10 or more reps for most
rowing exercises is recommended.

Wide-Grip Seated Row

Using a wide grip (ideally with neutral handles, but overhand grip is fine
also) can help beat shoulder glide at its own game, so to speak. A big body
blocking typical range of motion in a seated row needs only a very wide
hand position to make that same range of motion a much more natural stopping point to the movement. Similar to the way an ultra-wide-grip bench
press can reduce range of motion on the exercise to reach full extension,
applying the same logic to the seated row by using a pull-down bar and a
far distance between the hands results in a shorter range of motion to reach
full shoulder blade retraction. As long as the elbows remain in line with the
bar, this will also encourage the activity of more rear deltoids thanks to the
flared elbow position.

As far as the row itself goes, the same mechanics apply, including some
mild top rock and a neutral or slightly extended lumbar spine throughout the
entirety of the lift. The point of contact on the torso will inevitably be higher
up to respect alignment among the wrist, elbow, and shoulder, similar, once
again, to a bench press and hand width determining point of contact.

This movement is best performed with an overhand grip if not neutral,
since using an underhand grip typically exceeds the range of external rotation and supination the upper arm and wrist, respectively, need in order to
perform properly and pain free.

Rows: Long Legs, Short Torso

Although the seated row can prove beneficial to this particular body type (especially when coupled with longer arms), these proportions are also suited for the bent-over row and its variations. It can be difficult for a lifter with a far distance between torso and floor to find the ideal position when performing the bent-over row, often resulting in the athlete standing up a bit too much when lifting; this doesn't target the scapular muscles, since standing too tall will more closely mimic a shrug pattern for the upper traps rather than a row pattern for the upper and mid back.

Best Variation: Pendlay Row

Popularized by Glenn Pendlay, this bent-over row variation provides a necessary twist on the standard exercise. It halts the transfer of forces by creating a dead stop at the bottom of each rep. Removing this change of direction can reduce the amount of force the lumbar spine endures since the bar is given a chance to stop at the bottom, and the body is given crucial time to reset between reps.

This allows the lifter to focus on the concentric rep (pulling phase) more exclusively while remaining properly braced (figure 10.9a-b). Lifters who don't have the flexibility or mobility to pull from the floor with a flat back can raise the surface using low platforms, blocks, or plates to pull from, while ensuring the torso remains relatively parallel to the floor (figure 10.10a-b). All of this will give a lifter the capacity to pull the heaviest weight they can, while the erasure of momentum and energy transfer makes each rep much more honest and true to the extent of their actual ability, without being aided by kinetic forces.

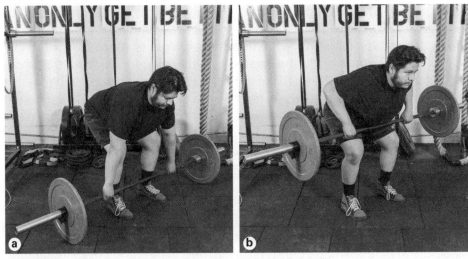

FIGURE 10.9   Pendlay row: start position (a), and finish (b).

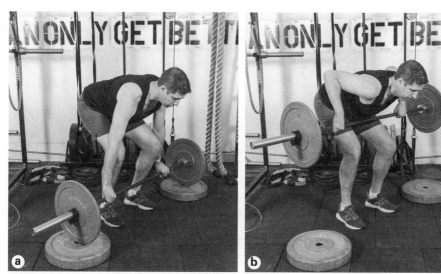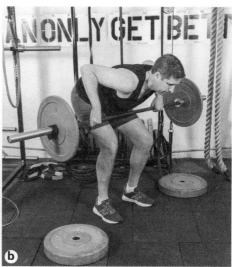

FIGURE 10.10 Modified Pendlay row: start on blocks *(a)*, and finish *(b)*.

The Pendlay row can be performed with an overhand or underhand grip, depending on mobility levels, comfort levels, and areas of the upper back a lifter wishes to target. Because of the loading and nature of the movement (and how similar in nature it is to a deadlift), lower rep ranges are appropriate. Sets of 6 to 8 reps are more desirable than sets of 12 to 15 reps, in order to better keep sets focused and for a lifter to take advantage of the opportunity to row heavier than normal weight for a concentric-biased pattern.

T-Bar Row

As mentioned earlier, classic bent-over rows can be a hassle for longer-legged lifters, since the common compensation is for the knees to start intersecting with the barbell's line of pull. It can be difficult to keep the bar clear of the knees on each repetition, and it is completely contingent on the lifter's maintaining a very hinged position at the hip, making for a parallel-to-floor torso position. Without a proper, full hinge and a parallel torso, a long-legged lifter will not be able to maintain vertical shins, and the torso will stay more upright than it should. Add to the fact that the lumbar spine deals with more forces while bearing load in this position (compared with a more upright torso position, as we broke down in chapter 5 when comparing barbell deadlifts to trap bar deadlifts), and it calls for a fresh look at force angles to ameliorate the situation and better target the upper back.

Using a T-bar for rows sets the load on an axis behind the body, rather than having 100 percent of the load in front of the legs (figure 10.11*a-b*). This changes the demand on the body and spine, since the fulcrum of the body (the hip joint) now has a more favorable distribution of load to bear—a third-class lever system; the force is produced in between the resistance and the fulcrum.

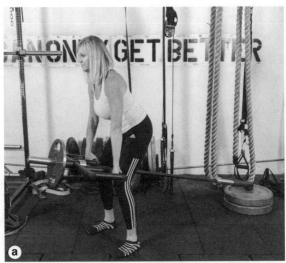

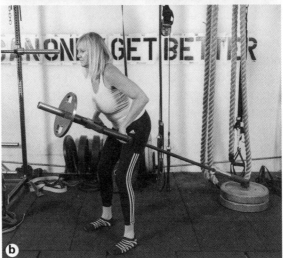

FIGURE 10.11   T-bar row: start position *(a)*, and finish *(b)*.

All of this, in addition to a nonlinear bar path thanks to the axis of the machine creating a smooth arcing pattern of the weight, means lower stresses on the spine and the ability to stand up taller while rowing, without a change to the physics of the movement as they pertain to upper back activity.

Most commonly, T-bars are front loaded, meaning weight plates are attached to a spot just in front of the handles of the machine. Occasionally, machines will have additional loading necks positioned behind the body, closer to the axis of the device. For lifters who have a history of back injury or lumbar pain, this setup would be desirable to further reduce the amount of load the lumbar spine will directly bear. Here, higher volume sets are less stressful on the spine than they are for a traditional bent-over row, since the body has access to the support it needs to sustain positioning for safe pulls.

Rows: Small Hands

Having smaller hands when performing any back isolation exercise can be upsetting for a lifter considering that grip strength often fatigues before the musculature of the upper back. It's difficult to achieve muscular development or strength gains when limited by how much one can hold, and smaller hands aren't friendly to circumferences of pulling objects, especially when they're not barbells. Rubber-coated pulling handles for rows can be thicker than for standard Olympic bars, which is doing no favors for a smaller-handed lifter.

For those reasons, lifting straps can come in handy (figure 10.12). The setup is slightly different from using straps for deadlifts. Since the row serves fewer overall purposes than a deadlift does (its main purpose is to isolate and develop the upper back musculature, while becoming more efficient at the pattern), it is less oriented toward maximum strength development and less neurologically taxing. (Most rowing variations are less compound in nature, involve less weight lifted, and involve fewer moving joints.) Training with straps allows a lifter to place more emphasis on the middle and upper back muscles while using the hands and arms as anchors rather than prime movers.

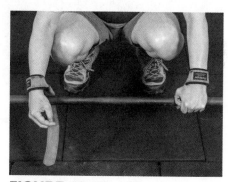

FIGURE 10.12 Lifting straps.

Band-Resisted Row

Using bands to change the resistance profile of a row pattern can benefit grip strength for two reasons. First, a band alone in the hand rather than a full bar or other handle will take up less surface area and be easier to hold for a prolonged period in and of itself. Second (and more importantly), the substitution from absolute weight to bands means the lifter doesn't need to deal with the same amount of loading through the entire force curve. As the arms fully extend, the resistance reduces itself since the bands are not as stretched, which makes it much easier for the lifter to attain and maintain proper form and technique through the whole movement; it is also much easier for the lifter to maintain grip since demand on the hands and forearms will be significantly lower for a portion of each rep (figure 10.13a-b). This can preserve forearm strength and delay fatigue, making it easier to maintain an intended focal point. Even if handles are attached to bands for a more ergonomic pull, the noted changes in the resistance profile will prove beneficial for small-handed lifters.

Although it's much more difficult to quantify the amount of weight lifted in the case of a banded exercise compared with a conventionally weighted movement, thicker bands or multiple bands can be used to present a greater challenge. Moreover, the amount of weight a lifter can move in an exercise like rows should be lower on the priority list than the quality of movement being produced, the hit received for the muscles of the upper back, and the induction of fatigue in the right places.

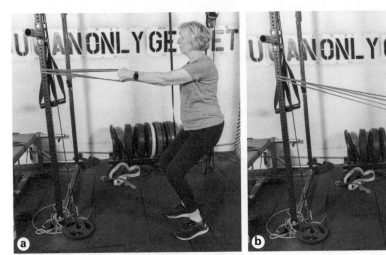

FIGURE 10.13 Band-resisted row: start position *(a)*, and finish *(b)*.

Row Patterns: Supplementary Movements

The row pattern in itself is typically viewed as a way to address issues within the body, especially the shoulder joint, because it's usually seen as something of a do-no-wrong exercise choice for healthy movement patterns and injury-free training. For that reason, there are no assistance exercises that would improve performance in the row pattern. With that said, certain mobility exercises, such as the foam roller thoracic extension explained in chapter 11, to ensure proper mechanics are being used when rowing can prove beneficial.

The row pattern is possibly the healthiest exercise in this book, as far as the reach it has toward improving posture, strengthening the shoulder joint, and maximizing shoulder function with the fewest drawbacks or risks attached to its frequent practice. For these reasons, it's a pattern that should be trained often. Many strength coaches recommend a 2:1 ratio of pull exercises to push exercises in a standard training workout, but we'll go a step further and recommend another ratio within the ratio just stated: 2:1 horizontal pulls (or rows) compared with overhead pulls. Following such a directive will ensure the shoulder joint gets safely trained and strengthened within a safe range of motion and joint angle. Moreover, the options aren't limited to one kind of row—a lifter can use whatever row patterns best suit them to get the job done; it's very difficult to overtrain the upper back. Use what we've shared in this chapter to select the best variations for your clients, and the thanks that will be delivered by way of improved pain-free performance and overall strength will be undeniable.

Chapter 11

Abdominal Stability

Abdominal stability is key in just about every athletic movement and sporting event. Any time the body lifts or carries an object, the abdominal, diaphragm, spinal, and pelvic floor muscles must brace to protect the integrity of the spine. There is no one dominant core stabilization muscle—all the muscles of the trunk work together to help stabilize the body (McGill et al. 2003).

Core stability is integral in maintaining posture and in resisting forces (as in anti-rotation or in keeping the body upright when forces are pulling it backward or forward). High levels of core stability mean less chance of the body buckling under pressure. When the stabilizers of the core are weak, the body is more prone to injury and pain (Wilson et al. 2015). It is therefore extremely important not only for lifters but for humans in general to maintain general core strength and stability.

Interestingly, injuries in the lower limbs can negatively affect the ability of the core to stabilize, and conversely, an unstable core can increase risk of injury in the lower limbs (Wilson et al. 2015). Core strength helps create a stable base of support for any movement and is a key player in just about every major lift mentioned in this book. Therefore, this book must include a chapter on the importance of core stability.

In this chapter, we discuss common issues in core stability often seen within different body leverage types and how these stabilization issues can be addressed.

Abdominal Stability: Big All Over

Big-all-over athletes may have some mobility issues when it comes to abdominal training. Torsos with larger circumferences, for instance, may get in the way of an athlete performing a full sit-up or any movement in which the knees would need to be closer to the torso. In addition, big-all-over athletes may find movements such as planks to be a challenge—a bigger torso may touch the floor in an elbow plank and may require alternative positioning—or the total weight of the athlete's torso may prove challenging to manage in extended plank-type exercises such as wheel rollouts or in hanging abdominal movements such as hanging leg raises. The following exercises may prove useful for larger athletes who have difficulty with traditional abdominal stability movements.

Thoracic Rotation

Having a large amount of muscle or a large body does not necessarily lead to a lack of mobility. However, it is not uncommon to see mobility difficulties, particularly in trunk rotation, with this body type. A simple test for assessing an athlete's thoracic rotation is the seated rotation test (Howe and Read 2015). In this assessment, the athlete sits on a chair. The angles of the athlete's hips and knees should be at 90 degrees, and the athlete should maintain a neutral spine. The athlete crosses their hands at their chest and holds a dowel across the elbows (figure 11.1a). Holding an approximately 8-inch (20 cm) ball between the knees to stabilize the pelvic area, the athlete rotates

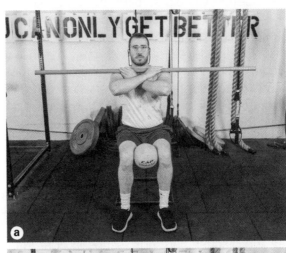

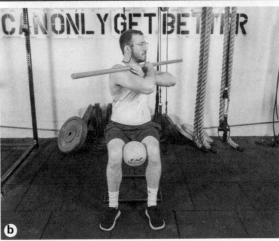

FIGURE 11.1   Rotation test: start *(a)*, and finish *(b)*.

to their end range in either direction (figure 11.1*b*). A goniometer—a simple device that measures the degree to which an object rotates—can be used to assess the degree of rotation achieved.

The degree of rotation needed for the athlete in question may deviate from the normal standard of about 55 degrees for a healthy nonathlete (Howe and Read 2015), so the requirements of the athlete's sport or activities should be considered. In addition, assessing and prescribing treatment for a thoracic mobility issue might be outside your scope of practice as a coach or trainer, so your capabilities and limitations should be considered. Refer out to a physical therapist or other medical professional where necessary.

Supine Spinal Rotation

Supine spinal rotation is a safe way to increase strength and mobility in thoracic rotation and is easily scaled up or down. The athlete lies on their back with arms out to the sides in line with the shoulders. The knees and hips will be at 90-degree angles, with the shins parallel to the floor (figure 11.2*a*). Without raising any part of the shoulders off the floor, and without changing the angle of the hips, the athlete slowly brings the knees to one side of the body as if to put them on the floor (figure 11.2*b*). Once end range of motion is reached, they slowly bring the knees back to center and repeat

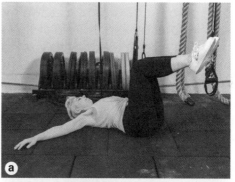
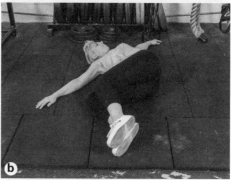
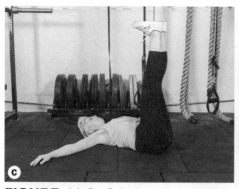
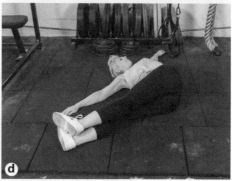

FIGURE 11.2 Spinal rotation with knees bent: start *(a)*, and finish *(b)*. Spinal rotation with knees straight: start *(c)*, and finish *(d)*.

on the other side. The athlete can make this movement more challenging by straightening the legs more (figure 11.2*c-d*). The straighter the legs, the more challenging the exercise.

Elongation Exercises

Bigger, heavier athletes may have difficulty maintaining the integrity of their spines in core movements that require elongating the body, such as wheel rollouts, extended plank exercises, and inchworms. Modifying these exercises to make them more manageable is key.

Foam Roller Thoracic Extensions

Lifters who suffer from excessive thoracic flexion would benefit from using a foam roller as a tool to aid in thoracic extension (figure 11.3). Lying with the foam roller placed widthwise across the mid-back allows the lifter to use the foam roller as a tactile cue to "wrap the back" around it. The lifter can simply lie back over the foam roller and achieve extension by allowing the back to stretch backwards over it. If it is more comfortable for the lifter, they can bring the hands behind the head to support the weight of the head. This exercise is more accessible to many lifters due to its passive nature, compared to the active nature of most thoracic spine extension drills.

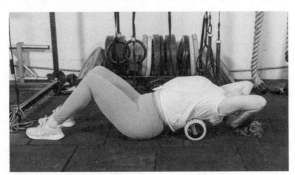

FIGURE 11.3   Foam roller thoracic extension.

Wheel Rollouts

In the wheel rollout, the athlete's pelvis should be tucked (in posterior tilt) so that the curve of the lower back is minimized and the abdominals are braced through the length of the exercise. A heavier athlete may find it very challenging to manage the weight of their body through longer ranges of motion in the rollout.

One way to modify wheel rollouts in order to reduce back strain for the bigger athlete is to station the athlete in front of a sturdy wall or door. The distance to the wall should be very slightly beyond the end point of the athlete's rollout ability, but at which the athlete can still maintain good form.

Rolling to the wall will keep the athlete from losing control of the movement and losing form and will strengthen the core at the end range of motion.

Band-assisted wheel rollouts are another option that can be very useful to the larger-bodied athlete (figure 11.4). In this modification, a stretch band is attached to the top of a squat cage or other sturdy area above the athlete. The other end of the stretch band is around the athlete's waist. The band will support the weight of the athlete as they perform the movement. The difficulty of this modification can be adjusted by changing the thickness of the bands—thicker bands will, of course, provide more support than thinner bands.

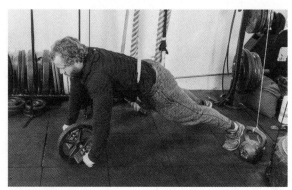

FIGURE 11.4   Band-assisted rollout.

Suspension Trainer Standing Rollout

Using a suspension trainer allows the athlete to manage the angle of the rollout, making it easier to control the movement. This exercise is particularly valuable for long-armed athletes and big-all-over athletes, who may find traditional rollouts to be unwieldy.

The athlete holds the handles of the suspension trainer and stands at an angle as if they are about to do a push-up. The hands are in line with the shoulders, and the ribs and hips are pulled toward each other to reduce the curve in the lower back and help stabilize the spine. Keeping the arms completely straight and their weight in their hands, the athlete slowly brings the arms up by their ears, as in a wheel rollout, and then returns to the starting position. The torso remains rigid throughout the exercise.

This movement can be made more or less challenging simply by walking the feet forward or backward. The more parallel the athlete gets to the floor, the more challenging this will be.

Inchworms

Inchworms, or hand walkouts, are an excellent substitute for wheel rollouts for heavier and for longer-limbed lifters. Inchworms help increase mobility in the lower back and hamstrings and give the lifter more control over the eccentric portion of the movement than they might with a wheel.

Keeping their legs as straight as their flexibility allows, the lifter places their hands on the floor in front of their feet (figure 11.5a). They then walk their hands forward until they are in a push-up position (figure 11.5b). It is important to keep the lower back as flat as possible to prevent any sagging of the spine in this exercise. If the lifter would like more of a challenge, they can continue to walk the hands as far forward as possible without letting the lower back drop.

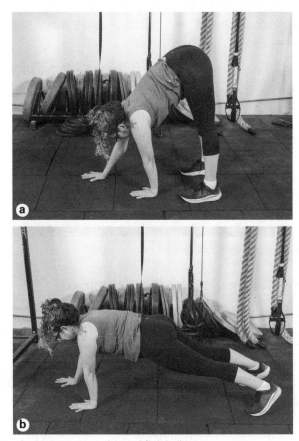

FIGURE 11.5   Inchworm: start (a), and finish (b).

Abdominal Stability: Long Arms

Having long arms can be a challenge in movements like wheel rollouts and extended plank positions—the longer levers make these positions more challenging to progress to full extension. Then again, we can also look at that as perhaps an advantage—if you can, in fact, achieve a full-extension wheel rollout with long arms and a long torso, you have likely got great core strength!

In abdominal stability exercises requiring arm extension, long-armed athletes can use their long levers to make movements significantly more challenging than they would be for shorter-armed athletes. They will also need to modify these movements as they are in the process of building that strength. This section provides a few exercises in which long arms can be used or reined in to modify the resistance.

Long-Arm Sit-Up

Having a long humerus can be an advantage in the military-style sit-up (in which the subject touches elbows to thighs with every repetition) (Dhayal 2020). This makes sense, since a longer upper arm has less distance to travel in order to bring the elbows to the thighs. Having long arms can also create an extra challenge in the sit-up where desired, by using the following modification.

This variation of the sit-up requires the athlete to hold their arms straight up overhead in line with the ears for the duration of the exercise (figure 11.6a). This makes the sit-up more challenging because the lever arm (the torso and extensions thereof) has been elongated (figure 11.6b). The longer the arms, the more challenging this movement can be. To make it even more challenging, the subject can hold a weight in the hands while performing the long-arm sit-up.

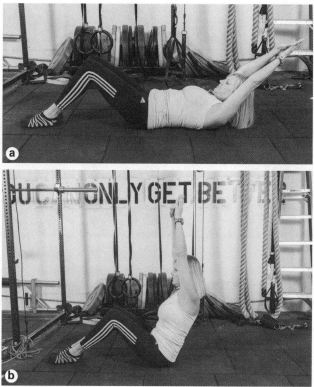

FIGURE 11.6   Long-arm sit-up: start (a), and finish (b).

Pallof Press

The Pallof press requires the lifter to stand parallel to the attachment point of a cable or elastic band (figure 11.7*a*). The lifter holds the handle or end of the band at the chest with both hands and then slowly extends the arms straight out to lockout, resisting the pull of the cable or band. The lifter then returns the hands to the chest and repeats for the desired number of reps. The idea is to keep the weight of the cable or band from perturbing the position of the torso.

The Pallof press can also be done vertically, with the cable or band in back of the athlete (so that the athlete is resisting being pulled backward), or laterally (figure 11.7*b-c*), with the cable or band above or below and beside the athlete (so that the athlete is resisting being pulled into a side bend). The movement can also be done from various lunging, squatting, and kneeling positions to further challenge the stability of the core and for sport-specific purposes.

Long arms can make this anti-rotation exercise and its variations more challenging because of the distance of the hands from the body at the end point of the movement. A longer-armed athlete may need lower weight than a shorter-armed athlete to successfully perform the Pallof press.

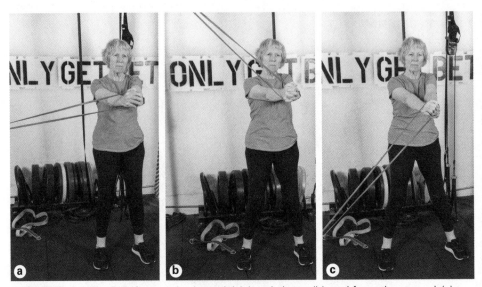

FIGURE 11.7   Pallof press: horizontal *(a)*, band above *(b)*, and from the ground *(c)*.

Abdominal Stability: Long Legs

Long legs can be a challenge when it comes to exercises involving lifting the legs, such as hanging leg raises, supine leg raising and lowering movements, and advanced calisthenic exercises such as flags and levers. Because longer legs encompass a larger percentage of the total body compared with the core, a longer-legged subject might employ compensatory movements that could put the lower back or hips at risk of injury in certain exercises.

Alternate Leg Lowering

Alternate leg lowering is an excellent exercise to build abdominal strength and stability for the long-legged athlete in particular. The athlete lies supine on the ground with the hips and knees at 90-degree angles (figure 11.8a). The lower back is pressed into the ground as much as possible. If desired, a partner can place a thin band or piece of paper underneath the athlete's lumbar spine and gently tug at it for the duration of this exercise to ensure the lower back is pressed into the ground. Without letting the spine come off the ground and without changing the hip angle of the opposite leg, the athlete slowly lowers one foot to the floor and then brings it back to the starting position. The movement is repeated on the opposite leg. As more strength is gained in this exercise, the knee angle can be slowly increased to increase the difficulty of the movement (figure 11.8b).

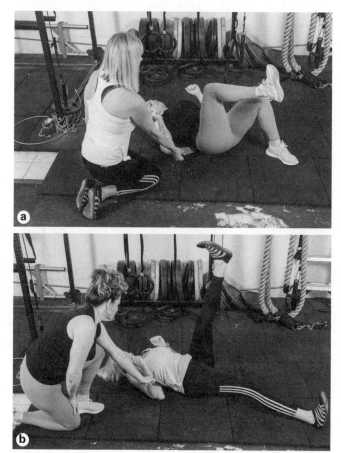

FIGURE 11.8   Alternate leg lowering: with bent knees (a), and straight knees (b).

Hanging Knee Raise

The long-legged athlete may have trouble doing toe-to-bar exercises. In this case, a hanging knee raise may be an appropriate alternative. The knee raise automatically decreases the lever length of the legs, making the exercise more manageable (figure 11.9a-b). As the athlete gains more strength in this movement, the angle of the knee may be increased incrementally in order to increase the difficulty of the exercise and further challenge the trunk muscles.

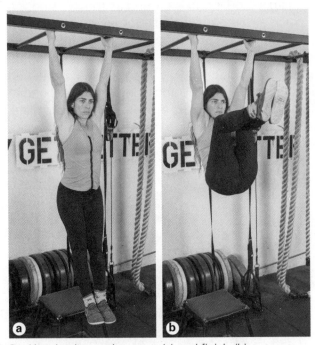

FIGURE 11.9   Hanging knee raise: start (a), and finish (b).

This strategy may also be used in similar types of exercises. In the side-to-side leg lowering exercise, for instance, the athlete begins in a supine position with the hips and knees both at a 90-degree angle and the arms directly out to the sides. The athlete then lowers the knees to one side of the body as low as possible, ensuring that the hip and knee angles do not change and the opposite shoulder does not come off the floor. The athlete then brings the legs back to center and over to the other side in the same way. As more strength is built in this exercise, the angle of the knees can slowly be increased.

Abdominal Stability: Small Hands

Smaller hands tend to be at a significant disadvantage in feats requiring gripping, such as deadlifts and pull-ups (Alahmari et al. 2017; Günther et al. 2008). Grip strength can also be predicted by the circumference of the forearm (Rice, Williamson, and Sharp 1998). Therefore, building forearm girth and hand strength is of particular interest to the smaller-handed athlete. Weighted carries can be an excellent tool to build grip strength as well as core strength for the small-handed lifter.

Weighted Carries

Weighted carries can be performed unilaterally or bilaterally, depending on the goals of the athlete. A single-handed weighted carry forces the spine to stabilize laterally more than a bilateral weighted carry and therefore may be a useful variation.

Any weighted implement can be used to perform the farmer's walk—dumbbells, kettlebells, hex bars, or specialized farmer's walk bars and frames all work well for this exercise (figure 11.10). Increasing the circumference of the handle can challenge the grip more. This can be achieved by wrapping a towel or shirt around the handle of the implement or by using a thick grip attachment or an apparatus with thicker handles.

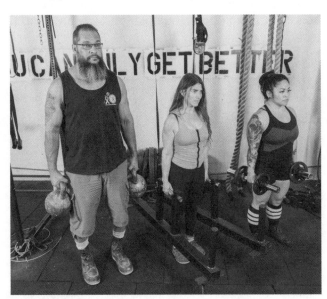

FIGURE 11.10   Weighted carries.

Hanging Abdominal Exercises and Grip Strength

Grip strength is an extremely important component of total body strength (if an athlete cannot hold on to the barbell, they're not going to be able to lift it!). To do hanging leg raises, the athlete must be able to hang from a bar for the duration of the exercise and be able to maintain the grip on the bar through changes in body position. With that in mind, one way to start building grip strength for these types of exercises is to practice hanging from a bar for as long as possible, slowly building up the hang time. Another option is to perform the hanging leg raises one or two repetitions at a time, then taking a quick break and doing another repetition or two. The athlete should try to increase the number of repetitions done in a row over time until they can all be performed without a rest in between.

Captain's Chair Exercise

For people whose grip is not strong enough to hang from a bar, or for lifters who simply want a different variation of the hanging leg raise, a captain's chair is a good alternative.

The captain's chair, also known as the Roman chair, is a padded device with two arm rests and a pad for the back, much like an armchair without the seat. In this exercise, the athlete places their elbows on the arm pads. The back should be straight and braced against the back pad, and the shoulders should be pushed down and away from the ears so that the athlete is not sagging or shrugging during the exercise (figure 11.11a). Once in position,

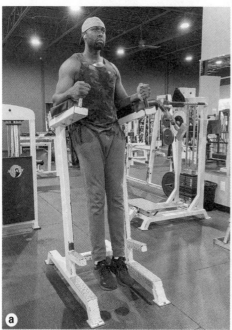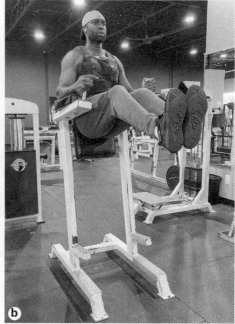

FIGURE 11.11   Captain's chair: start *(a)*, and finish *(b)*.

the athlete performs the hanging leg raise in much the same way as when hanging from a bar—raise and lower the knees (or straight legs, for an advanced version) as high as possible without swinging or otherwise using momentum (figure 11.11b).

Decline Leg Raise

One issue with a captain's chair is that the arms are fixed and not adjustable for different body types. As such, people with shorter arms may find it very uncomfortable and may not be able to position their arms optimally. For those athletes, a decline leg raise may be an ideal hybrid between a hanging leg raise and a captain's chair exercise. The decline leg raise can also be a useful exercise for any athlete whose grip is not yet strong enough to do a hanging leg raise, or simply as an alternative exercise to the hanging leg raise.

The decline leg raise requires the athlete to use a decline bench with an attachment at the top that the user can hold on to securely (a handle, a leg attachment, or some similar addition). The athlete sets the bench at the desired angle (the steeper the angle, the harder the movement) and lies on the bench on their back, head resting on the higher portion of the bench (figure 11.12a). While holding the top attachment tightly with both hands, the athlete tries to bring the legs toward the chest and back to the starting position (figure 11.12b). The buttocks and lower back will come off the bench and curl toward the chest in this movement. Momentum should not be used at any point in the exercise.

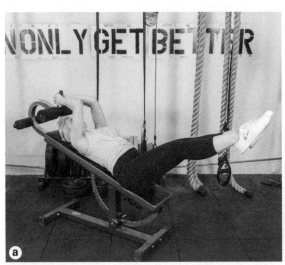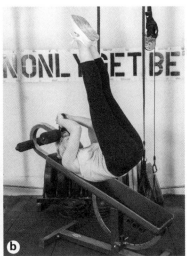

FIGURE 11.12 Decline bench leg raise: start (a), and finish (b).

Additional Intermediate Options for Core Training

This section offers some effective alternative exercises for training the core.

Mountain Climber

Mountain climbers provide excellent conditioning benefits while also helping to strengthen the abdominals, lower back, core, hips, and legs. They may also help increase levels of coordination and flexibility over time. A mountain climber is essentially a high plank during which the legs perform a running-like movement. The athlete puts their hands about shoulder-width apart on the ground, keeping the arms completely straight. The body should be in a plank position, with the hips in line with the head and toes, the head in a neutral position, and the abdominals braced so that the lower back does not sag (figure 11.13a). The athlete drives one knee toward the same-side arm as quickly as possible, placing the toe on the floor (figure 11.13b-c). Then the athlete returns that leg back to the start position and immediately repeats the movement with the opposite leg. It is very important to keep the body in plank position for the duration of the movement; the athlete should not lift the hips or drop the lower back.

Athletes who are big all over may encounter mobility challenges in this movement, and athletes with long legs and short arms may have difficulty clearing the floor properly throughout this exercise. For those athletes who find traditional mountain climbers overly challenging or who cannot perform them with good form, placing the hands on an elevated object such as yoga blocks or a sturdy bench might be a preferable alternative.

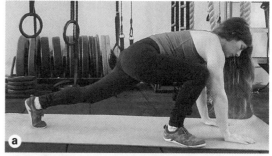

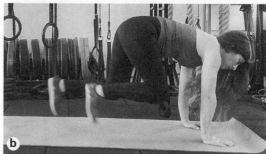

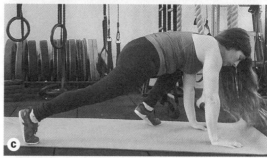

FIGURE 11.13 Mountain climber: start position (a) middle (b), and finish (c).

Chinese Plank

The Chinese plank is an anti-flexion exercise that can be performed in a prone position or supine position. The supine version of the Chinese plank helps to strengthen the entire posterior chain from the shoulders to the feet. The prone version helps to strengthen the abdominals, hip flexors, quadriceps, and spine. Both versions of the Chinese plank can be performed on their own or can be used as a base position from which to perform barbell or dumbbell movements such as the bench press or row.

Supine Chinese Plank

In the supine version of the Chinese plank (figure 11.14a), the athlete places a bench or box under the head and upper shoulders and places another box or bench of equal height under the heels. The athlete then squeezes the glutes, locks the legs, and braces the abdominals so that the body is completely rigid and in a straight line. The resulting position should essentially look like a good standing position.

Prone Chinese Plank

In the prone Chinese plank (figure 11.14b), the athlete places a box or bench under the shoulders and places another box or bench of equal height under the toes. The athlete then braces the abdominals, squeezes the glutes, and locks the legs to achieve a horizontal standing-like position. To avoid discomfort due to head and neck placement, the lifter may place the upper body bench so that the chin extends over the edge of the bench, or they may choose to use three benches for the upper body, with one under each shoulder and one under the

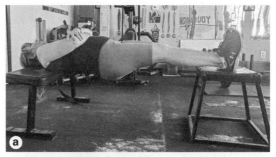
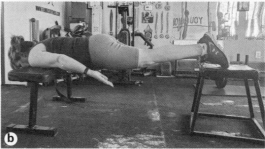

FIGURE 11.14 Chinese plank: supine (a), and prone (b).

toes. Women may prefer this three-bench version if there is discomfort when putting pressure on the chest.

Taller athletes typically find the Chinese plank more challenging because there is more body length to hold stable. To decrease the difficulty of the plank, the benches for the upper body and feet can be placed closer together. To increase the difficulty, the athlete can wear a weighted vest or place a weight on the torso.

Breathing

Breathing is of utmost importance for all lifting. Breathing properly helps oxygenate the blood and can help brace the abdominals, creating an inner weight belt of sorts. There is some evidence that holding the breath during lifting causes the blood pressure to rise significantly, although more and higher-quality research is needed in order to confirm this theory (Perkilis 2019).

Diaphragmatic breathing (i.e., breathing into the stomach) is a way to fill the lungs completely with air and create pressure and tension throughout the lower abdominal region in order to better support a heavy weight or resist a force. One way to learn proper breathing technique is for the lifter to lie on their abdomen on the ground, hands under the forehead to support the head more comfortably in this position. The lifter will then breathe in through the nose, concentrating on "pushing the floor away" with the lower abdominals.

Another method to practice this type of breathing is to lie on the back and place one hand on the chest and another on the lower abdominal region. When the lifter breathes in through the nose, the shoulders should not elevate, and only the hand on the lower abdominals should feel movement.

In a heavy lift or bracing situation, on the breath out, the lifter places the tongue behind the teeth and breathes out forcefully in order to press the diaphragm down. This movement should push the abdomen out as well, creating a stable core to support the lift. This breath out occurs on the most challenging part of the lift (the pressing motion in the bench press, for instance, or the upward portion of the squat).

The muscles of the trunk should never be neglected, and it's fitting that this chapter occurs later in the book rather than earlier to properly establish context and pull things together. Because the spine is arguably the number one area of the body requiring protection, it's important that a combination of proper technique, proper breathing, correct bracing, and of course, the right supplementary exercises (especially for a given body type) be employed to ensure safety and amplify gains. The trunk is a region of the body that lifters tend to neglect to train in specificity. However, especially if a lifter has a history of injury to the spine or surrounding tissue, it's a weak link that demands attention, and its development as a unit is key—just like every other part of the body.

PART III

Rounding Out a Comprehensive Strength Program

We have discussed general exercise guidelines for the big movements. In this section, we will discuss the fine-tuning of those movements. Just as the adjustment of the bigger movements (and any exercise prescription, really) has a lot of nuance and no hard-and-fast rules, the ways in which those movements can be strengthened and developed into a program specific to an athlete are also highly variable. It cannot be emphasized enough that every body is different. Even within body type categories, individual bodies will have different goals, abilities, and structures. There can never be rigid recommendations where the human body is concerned.

That said, in this section, we will provide suggestions for accessory movements that may help improve strength in the big lifts. While there are recommendations that would be useful in a general sense for weaknesses that may appear within particular body types, these movements can be selected based on individual needs.

Chapter 12

Accessory Work

The primary exercises discussed in this book are the deadlift, squat, bench press, overhead press, chin-up, and row. Those chapters include several variations of each exercise that can help improve performance for different body leverage types.

Accessory exercises are the movements that fill out the rest of the workout and target weak points to make the primary lifts stronger. Accessory exercises tend not to use as much weight as major lifts and are often performed for more repetitions. They can be single-joint exercises, such as triceps extensions and leg curls, or multiple-joint exercises such as diamond push-ups. This chapter describes a variety of accessory exercises that may be of particular benefit for the primary movements described in this book.

Considerations for Upper Body Pressing Exercises

As noted earlier in this book, the triceps are an extremely important component of pressing exercises. For long-armed individuals in particular, strengthening the triceps may make the difference in locking out a heavy load. Many training programs include single-joint triceps exercises such as kickbacks, triceps press-downs, and so forth in order to strengthen this muscle. A number of studies have demonstrated that single-joint movements in conjunction with multiple-joint movements do not improve performance (Barbalho et al. 2018; de Franca et al. 2015; Gentil, Fisher, and Steele 2017).

The effectiveness of single-joint movements should not be ruled out, however. The previously mentioned studies were both short term and small, and more research needs to be done before drawing conclusions on this subject. Training single-joint exercises may help overcome muscle imbalances, may provide sport-specific advantages, can allow the joints in question to move through ranges of motion not possible in a multiple-joint exercise, and may be useful for injury prevention and recovery (Schoenfeld and Contreras 2012). Single-joint movements may also improve muscle hypertrophy (de Franca et al. 2015; Mannarino et al. 2021). Bigger arms may lead to bigger presses, so hypertrophy can contribute to pressing strength.

That said, including both single- and multiple-joint accessory movements that target the triceps may be useful not only for improving pressing performance but also for adding variety to a pressing program. Variety helps prevent repetitive stress issues that may result from bench pressing or military pressing several times per week.

Single-Joint Triceps Exercises

The amount each head of the triceps is activated seems to change depending on the height of the elbow in relation to the shoulder (Kholinne et al. 2018). At a 0-degree angle, the long head of the triceps is the dominant portion. As the elbow is brought upward, the medial head of the triceps becomes the main force in extending the elbow. Therefore, performing single-joint triceps extensions at varying angles may target different parts of the triceps.

Best Practice for Bench Press: Tate Press

The Tate press is a single-joint triceps extension that mimics the lockout position in the bench press. Because of its general specificity to the bench press movement, it can be a very useful exercise for improving bench press performance.

The lifter lies on their back on the bench, arms locked, palms facing away from the head, holding two dumbbells straight above the chest as in the top of a dumbbell bench press (figure 12.1a). Bending the elbows laterally, the lifter lowers the dumbbells toward the middle of the chest and then presses the dumbbells back up again to the start position (figure 12.1b).

Big-all-over lifters may not achieve as much benefit from the Tate press as other lifters might, since the range of motion in which the dumbbells travel

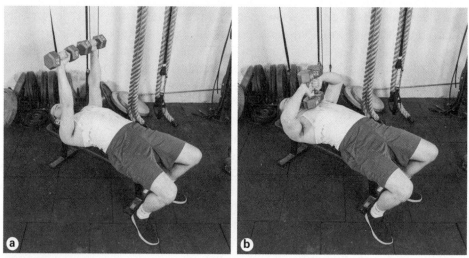

FIGURE 12.1   Tate press: start *(a)*, and finish *(b)*.

will be shortened because of the height of the lifter's chest. However, the movement mimics the general range of motion of the lifter's bench press, and so it may still be useful.

Best Practice for Overhead Press: Overhead Triceps Extension

Overhead triceps extensions place the elbow above the shoulder, therefore targeting the medial head of the triceps in particular (Kholinne et al. 2018). The overhead triceps extension can be performed unilaterally or bilaterally and has sport-specific applications for overhead throwing athletes. We recommend performing this movement unilaterally because this prevents the dominant arm from overpowering the exercise; it also allows for some freedom of movement in the angle of the hand, wrist, and arm, therefore lowering the risk of elbow pain during the exercise. Performed standing, the overhead triceps extension can also challenge core stability as well as shoulder stability.

The single-arm overhead triceps extension can be performed with a dumbbell, kettlebell, cable, or band. The lifter holds the weighted implement of their choice straight above their head (figure 12.2a). The lifter then slowly lowers the weight behind the head until they feel a substantial stretch in the triceps area, then extends the elbow to the start position without moving the upper arm (figure 12.2b).

Ideally, the upper arm will remain close to the head and perpendicular to the floor. However, some athletes may not have the flexibility to place their arm in this position. If that is the case, the lifter can just keep the elbow at the highest height possible without pain. Lifters with especially large upper arm circumference may not be able to get as much range of motion as lifters with a smaller upper arm. In addition, longer arms may require lighter weights for the overhead triceps extension.

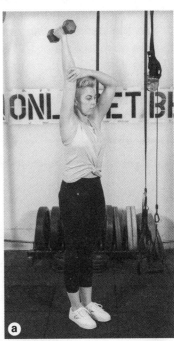

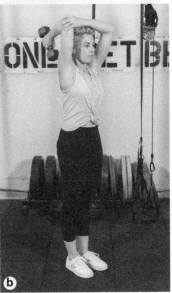

FIGURE 12.2 Single-arm overhead triceps extension: start (a), and finish (b).

Triceps Press-Down

The triceps press-down is done with no flexion of the shoulder and therefore is an excellent exercise to focus on the long head of the triceps (Kholinne et al. 2018). This movement is generally performed with a cable apparatus, although it can also be done with stretch bands. Press-downs can be performed unilaterally or bilaterally. As with the overhead triceps extension, we recommend a unilateral approach in order to train the arms with equal effort.

Set the cable or band at a point above the lifter's head. Grabbing the handle of the cable or the band, the lifter holds the elbow tight against the ribs as if they are holding a book under their arm (figure 12.3a). The lifter then straightens the arm at the elbow, without moving the upper arm, until the elbow is fully extended (figure 12.3b). Then the lifter slowly bends the arm back to the starting position and repeats as desired.

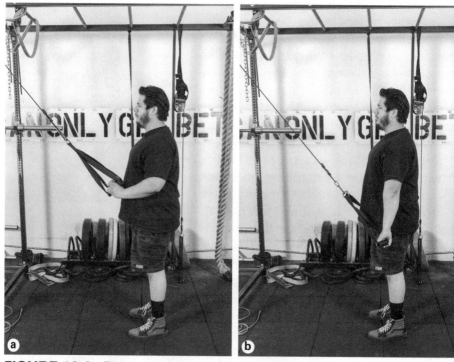

FIGURE 12.3   Triceps press-down: start (a), and finish (b).

Multiple-Joint Triceps Exercises

Multiple-joint accessory exercises such as push-ups can generally be done for many more repetitions than a heavy primary exercise such as a bench press. Push-ups can also be a primary exercise if the intention is to increase push-up performance. For the purposes of this book, the push-up is used as an accessory exercise to improve performance in pressing movements.

By changing the hand or body position of the movement, the push-up can easily be modified to emphasize different muscle combinations.

JM Press

Invented by elite bench press athlete J.M. Blakely, the JM press is a bench-press-specific, triceps-focused movement. In the JM press, the lifter starts lying supine on a bench while holding a barbell with arms straight over the shoulders, as in a bench press (figure 12.4a). They lower the bar toward the forehead as if to do a skull crusher. At the same time, the lifter brings the upper arms in line with the torso so they are as parallel to the floor as possible (figure 12.4b). The lifter then pushes the bar back to the starting position and repeats as necessary. The JM press is an interesting hybrid of the skull crusher and narrow-grip bench press, and it can be a very effective movement to improve triceps strength in the bench press.

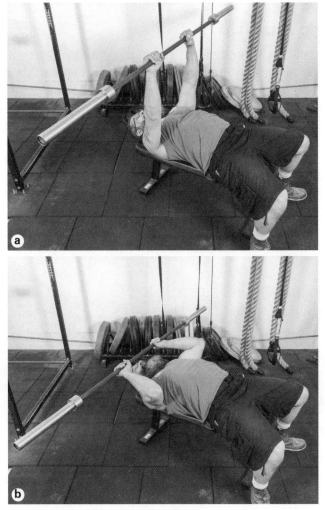

FIGURE 12.4   JM press: start (a), and finish (b).

Push-Ups

It appears that push-ups can be used interchangeably with the bench press—they have extremely similar movement geometry and muscle activation (van den Tillaar 2019). The basic push-up can be thought of as a moving plank—the torso should remain rigid without any sagging of the lower back or elevation of the hips. The hands are placed under or just outside of the shoulders. The elbows, when bent, should be at about 45 degrees from the ribs. The body should be lowered under control until it is as close to the floor as possible, and the hands then push into the floor and the arms straighten to bring the body back to the start position. The body moves as a unit in the push-up—no segment should be lowered or raised before any other segment.

There is a great deal of variety in hand placement, foot placement, and body movements within the push-up family, thus allowing lifters to train at many different angles and challenge themselves in different ways.

Plyometric Push-Up

Plyometric push-ups improve force production, which can have big payoffs when it comes to pressing heavier weight off the chest in a bench press. In a plyometric push-up, the athlete begins in tall plank position, with the hands under the shoulders, the arms locked at the elbow, the abdominals braced, and the torso in a straight line from head to ankles (i.e., no raising of the hips or sagging of the midsection). The athlete bends the elbows at a 45-degree angle from the ribs until the torso touches the floor (figure 12.5a). They then push the hands hard into the floor and try to "jump" off the floor with the hands as high as possible (figure 12.5b). When the hands return to

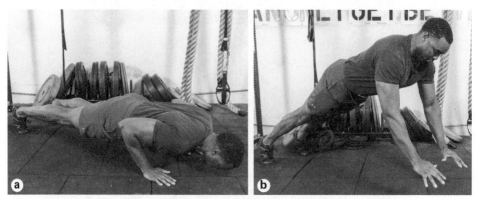

FIGURE 12.5   Plyometric push-up: start *(a)*, and finish *(b)*.

Extending the Depth of Push-Ups

Placing the hands on hex dumbbells, blocks, or push-up handles will increase the range of motion. Whereas the torso is stopped by the floor in a regular push-up, when the hands are up on blocks or handles (figure 12.6*a*), the torso has room to drop significantly lower (figure 12.6*b*). Push-ups can also be performed with the hands on unstable objects such as medicine balls to challenge the stability of the upper body.

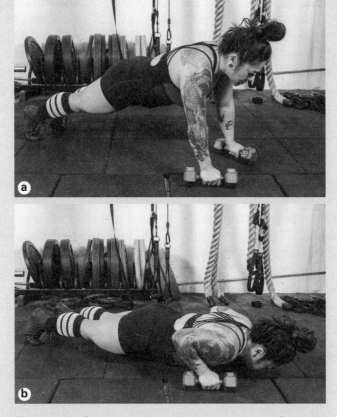

Figure 12.6   Push-up with dumbbells: start *(a)*, and finish *(b)*.

the floor, the athlete should bend the elbows and lower the torso to the floor again, repeating the movement. The athlete should never land with locked elbows, just as they should never jump and land on locked legs. The torso should remain in the rigid plank position for the duration of the movement.

Narrow- and Wide-Stance Push-Up

Of all push-up positions, the narrow-stance push-up targets the triceps the most (Kim, Kim, and Ha 2016; Marcolin et al. 2015), with shoulder-width positioning taking the second place position. In the narrow version, the hands are placed at about 50 percent of shoulder width and the push-up is otherwise performed as usual—the torso is rigid and in a straight line from head to feet, arms locked out in a tall plank in the starting position. The body is lowered under control until it touches the floor (or the hands). The athlete then pushes the body back to the tall plank position and repeats as desired.

The wide-stance push-up, performed as just described but with the hands wider than shoulder width, requires less effort from the triceps and pectorals and more work from the serratus anterior, biceps, and latissimus dorsi (Kim, Kim, and Ha 2016).

Push-ups of all kinds can be made less challenging by elevating the upper body so that less weight is on the hands. They can be made more challenging by adding a weighted vest or placing a weight plate on the back of the lifter.

Dips

Triceps dips are a multiple-joint exercise that can be integrated into a bench press program to strengthen both the triceps and the pectoral muscles. It should be noted that the end range of the dip exercise is a particularly vulnerable position for injury and may be a high-risk movement (McKenzie et al. 2021). Make sure the athlete performs dips within a pain-free range of motion and with excellent control of the exercise. If shoulder instability or pain is present, or if there are any concerns about shoulder impingement, it is recommended that the athlete select a different triceps exercise (diamond push-ups, for instance, may be a good substitution for dips).

Bench Dip

The bench dip is performed with the hands on a bench and the feet on the floor. The athlete's torso should be as vertical as possible, lined up directly underneath the shoulders. The shoulders are pressed down and back, away from the athlete's ears. Hunching the shoulders forward should be avoided. The athlete bends the arms to lower the body as much as possible and then pushes the arms back into the bench to straighten them and resume the starting position. The athlete can keep the knees bent at 90 degrees with the feet flat on the floor for an easier version of the bench dip (figure 12.7a) or can straighten the legs for a more challenging version (figure 12.7b). Bench dips can also be made more challenging by elevating the feet on another bench or chair (figure 12.7c) and by placing weight plates on the thighs.

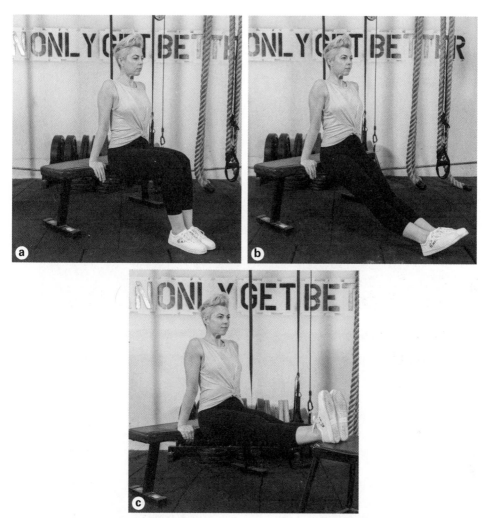

FIGURE 12.7   Bench dip with bent knees *(a)*, straight legs *(b)*, and elevated feet *(c)*.

Vertical Dip

In the vertical dip, the athlete begins with their hands on a set of parallel bars or a dip machine, arms locked out, shoulders depressed, and body suspended in the air (figure 12.8*a* and 12.8*c*). The athlete bends the elbows and leans forward (figure 12.8*b* and 12.8*d*), lowering their body as much as possible (ideally until the shoulders are lower than the elbows). The athlete then pushes into the bars to straighten the arms and resume the initial position, repeating as needed. The vertical dip can be made more challenging by adding a weighted vest or by attaching extra weight to a weight belt.

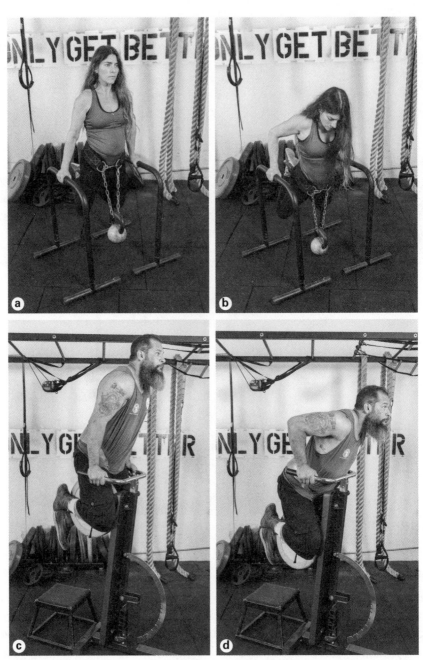

FIGURE 12.8 Vertical dip with weight belt on parallel bars: start *(a)*, and finish *(b)*. Vertical dip on dip machine: start *(c)*, and finish *(d)*.

The vertical dip appears to activate both the triceps brachii and the pectoralis major significantly more than does the basic bench dip (Bagchi 2015). However, positioning is important, and the pectoralis may be activated more in the vertical dip the more the athlete leans forward in the exercise. More challenging versions of the bench dip may also have differing effects on triceps activation.

Long-armed athletes may find vertical dips more challenging because of the longer distance they need to travel in this exercise. Big-all-over athletes may find vertical dips challenging as well, because they generally have more body weight to lift than smaller athletes. Athletes who struggle with vertical dips may choose to start with bench dips and build up strength from there, or they may choose an alternative exercise in order to minimize risk of shoulder injury.

Shoulder Accessory Exercises

Flys are movements in which the arms are extended to their full length and the shoulder becomes the fulcrum at the desired angle. Because the arms are extended in a fly, far less weight is needed to make these movements challenging than in a multiple-joint exercise such as a press.

Dumbbell and Machine Flys

Dumbbell and machine flys are as effective for pectoralis activation as the bench press (Welsch, Bird, and Mahew 2012). The time of activation is considerably shorter in the fly than in the press, however, so they are not a substitute for the press. That said, flys can be excellent accessory movements for gaining size and strength in the chest and anterior deltoids. Longer-armed athletes may need to use lighter weights than shorter-armed athletes in any movement that positions the weights farther from the body. Therefore, it is best for a longer-armed athlete to err on the side of lighter weights for flys and cable crossovers, and increase accordingly.

The dumbbell fly is performed by lying supine on a bench or on the floor. The lifter holds two dumbbells straight up above the chest, palms facing each other (figure 12.9a). Keeping a very slight bend in the elbow, the lifter lowers the arms straight out to the sides until the arms are in line with the shoulders (figure 12.9b). The lifter then reverses the movement until the arms are back at the initial position and repeats as desired.

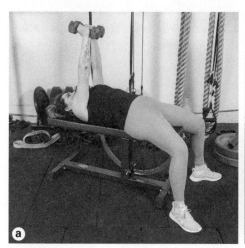 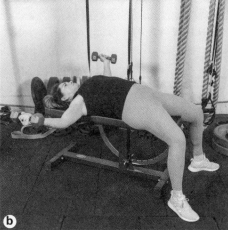

FIGURE 12.9 Dumbbell fly: start (a), and finish (b).

Cable Crossover

The cable crossover can also be performed in lieu of a dumbbell or machine fly. One benefit of the cable crossover is that the cables can be set at different angles, therefore challenging the deltoids and pectorals in different ways. The basic cable crossover is performed similarly to the fly. To start, the lifter stands in the center of the cable machine, halfway between the two pulleys. Holding one handle in each hand, the athlete steps forward a bit so the machine's weights elevate slightly off the stack (figure 12.10a). Some lifters prefer to stand with their feet staggered, while others prefer to stand with their feet parallel to each other; either method works as long as the lifter feels stable.

The athlete maintains a very slight bend in each arm. The arms always follow the path of the cables, so if the pulleys are in a low position, the arms will start in a low position and finish at chest height. If the cables are at shoulder height, the arms will travel in a straight line to chest height (figure 12.10b). If the cables are in a high position, the arms will travel downward and finish at about hip or navel height. In all cases, the athlete maintains the very slightly bent arm position and then returns the arms under control to the starting position.

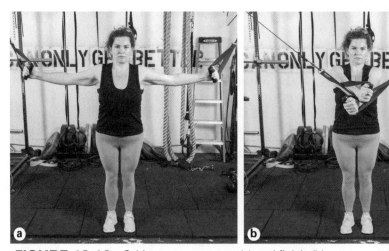

FIGURE 12.10   Cable crossover: start (a), and finish (b).

Cuban Press

The Cuban press is typically used as a dynamic warm-up exercise for the shoulders. It can be a useful movement for athletes with rotator cuff pain or shoulder instability, and it can help improve shoulder mobility.

The Cuban press is initiated with the athlete holding two dumbbells at their sides. The athlete shrugs the shoulders and elevates the elbows so the

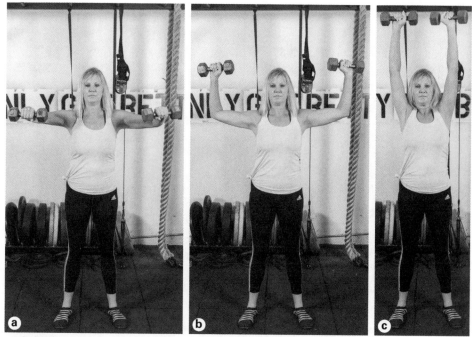

FIGURE 12.11   Cuban press: start *(a)*, middle *(b)*, and finish *(c)*.

upper arms are level with the shoulders (figure 12.11*a*). The lifter rotates the forearms until they are perpendicular to the floor (figure 12.11*b*), then presses the weights straight up as in a dumbbell military press (figure 12.11*c*). The Cuban press can also be performed the same way but in a bent-over position, or with the athlete lying prone on a bench, to challenge the posterior chain more. This movement should be done using very light weights—there is no need to try to maximize the load in the Cuban press.

Dumbbell Lateral Raise

The dumbbell lateral raise is a good way to build strength and stability in the shoulders in a nonpressing movement. It can help strengthen the shoulders in a range of motion not often trained in a pressing routine and can therefore be useful to help avoid repetitive stress injuries.

Holding two lighter dumbbells at their sides, the athlete keeps their arms almost completely locked (figure 12.12*a*). (A very small unlock of the elbow is fine.) The athlete raises their arms straight out to the sides, with the palms down, until their arms are in line with their shoulders (figure 12.12*b*). The athlete then slowly lowers the dumbbells and repeats as needed.

The longer the athlete's arms, the more challenging this movement can be, so weights should be selected accordingly. The lateral raise can also be performed with different hand positions (palms facing forward, palms facing up, or thumbs pointing down), depending on the needs of the athlete.

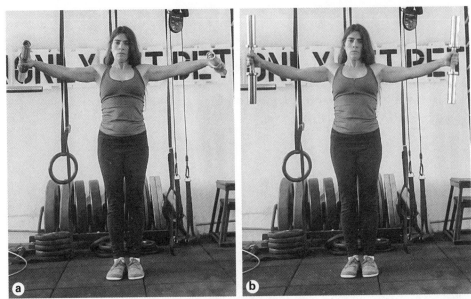

FIGURE 12.12   Dumbbell lateral raise: palms facing down *(a)*, and palms facing out *(b)*.

Considerations for Upper Body Pulling Exercises

Pulling exercises require a great deal of work from the muscles of the back, the biceps, and the forearm and hands. Just as single-joint and multiple-joint movements can be beneficial for pressing exercises, both types of movements can be equally important for improving pulling strength. Pulling exercises can also indirectly improve bench press performance. While it's up for debate exactly how much the latissimus dorsi contribute to bench press strength, having a bigger back will certainly add to the size of the torso, which, as we know, decreases the length of the bar path. This is particularly useful for lifters with longer arms, where shortening the bar path as much as possible is beneficial.

Single-Joint Biceps Exercises

Biceps strength plays an important role in pulling and carrying exercises, or in any movement requiring bending at the elbow. Single-joint biceps movements not only strengthen the muscles that flex the elbow joint but also play an important role in upper arm hypertrophy.

Biceps Curls

Biceps curls are the ultimate gym activity, and the one most people are familiar with regardless of experience. That said, biceps curls can be useful for both pressing and pulling exercises. They can help increase muscle mass (Mannarino et al. 2021), which is beneficial for pressing exercises. They are also specific to pulling exercises, since pulling requires elbow flexion.

Biceps curls can be done with a variety of apparatuses—barbells, dumbbells, cables, stretch bands, and so forth. For most standing varieties of biceps curls, the lifter starts by holding the dumbbells at their sides. Without moving the upper arm, the lifter bends the elbows to bring the dumbbells up toward the shoulders and then lowers the dumbbells back to the start position. There are a number of variations on this theme.

Standard Barbell Curl

Barbell curls generally allow for the most weight to be used in a curl exercise since both arms work together to lift one implement. However, a straight barbell fixes the hands in a completely supinated position, which some athletes find uncomfortable or painful. In addition, in a barbell curl, the stronger arm may end up taking on more work than the weaker arm. In a standard barbell curl, the hands are supinated for the duration of the exercise.

Standard Dumbbell Curl

Dumbbells allow for more freedom of movement of the hands and wrists to accommodate the needs of the lifter. Like the standard barbell curl, the palms face up for the entirety of the movement in a standard dumbbell curl.

Standard EZ-Bar Curl

An EZ-bar curl is another option; the bar's angled handle allows for a more comfortable wrist position for many people. In the standard version of the EZ-bar curl, the palms remain supinated for the entire movement.

Hammer Curl

In the hammer, or neutral-grip, curl, the dumbbells are held sideways, with the thumb side of the hand facing up on the curl (figure 12.13, right). Hammer curls can place less strain on the wrists than standard biceps curls, so they can be a good option to reduce repetitive stress from frequent performance of biceps curls, or for athletes who have pain or discomfort when performing standard curls.

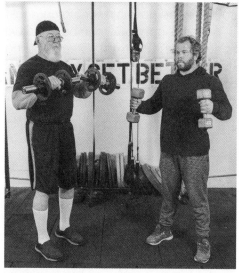

FIGURE 12.13 Hammer curl hand position (right) and reverse curl hand position (left).

Reverse Curl

In the reverse curl, the hands are pronated for the duration of the exercise to place the focus on forearm strength (figure 12.13, left). Both neutral-grip and pronated-grip biceps curls activate the brachioradialis, an elbow flexor in the forearm, more strongly than do standard curls (Boland, Spigelman, and Uhl 2008).

Zottman Curl

In the Zottman curl, the hands are supinated on the concentric portion of the movement, rotated at the top, and pronated on the eccentric portion of the movement. This exercise targets the forearms during the eccentric part of the movement.

Multiple-Joint Biceps Exercises

Multi-joint accessory exercises can be effective for building strength and hypertrophy for not only the targeted muscles, but also for the surrounding musculature. A bent-over row, for instance, will help strengthen the biceps, but also the rear deltoids and back muscles. Multi-joint accessory movements can build strength as well as single joint movements (Gentil, et al., 2015), and can serve as a way to mimic pushing and pulling patterns while providing enough variety to help reduce repetitive stress on the joints.

Reverse-Grip Bent-Over Row

The reverse-grip row targets the biceps a bit more than the standard row and also works the muscles of the upper and lower back as well as the rear deltoids. The reverse grip allows for a more powerful contraction of the biceps, so it may be possible for a bigger load to be pulled than in a traditional row.

Reverse-grip rows can be done with a barbell or with dumbbells. If there is discomfort with the fixed hand position in the barbell reverse-grip row, dumbbells or kettlebells are recommended. Furthermore, performing the reverse-grip row with dumbbells permits a greater range of motion than a barbell will allow.

Angle of Performance of Biceps Curls

The angle of the arms can also be changed. The arms can be pointed out to the sides, for example, or at a forward angle—as in the preacher curl (figure 12.14*a* and 12.14*b*), in which the upper arms are placed on an angled bench, or the spider curl (figure 12.14*c* and 12.14*d*), in which the athlete lies prone on an incline bench—and the curls are performed with the upper arms perpendicular to the floor. The shoulder can also be placed in a more extended position, as in the incline curl (figure 12.14*e* and 12.14*f*).

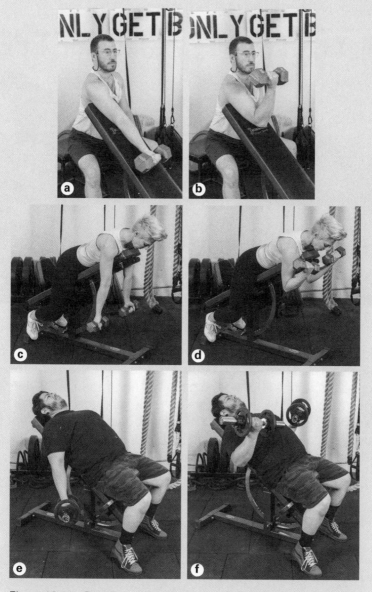

Figure 12.14   Preacher curl: start *(a)*, and finish *(b)*. Spider curl: start *(c)*, and finish *(d)*. Incline curl: start *(e)*, and finish *(f)*.

Varying the type of biceps curl performed can reduce repetitive stress on the elbow joint and change which portion of the elbow flexors is dominant in the exercise (Barakat et al. 2019).

The reverse-grip row is performed with the body in deadlift position, head neutral, spine rigid and slightly arched, hips back and high (but not higher than the head), and shins as perpendicular to the floor as possible (figure 12.15a). The barbell (or dumbbells or kettlebells) are held with the palms facing away from the body. The lifter pulls the elbows backward and toward each other, pulling the load all the way to the torso (figure 12.15b). The weight is then lowered back to the starting position.

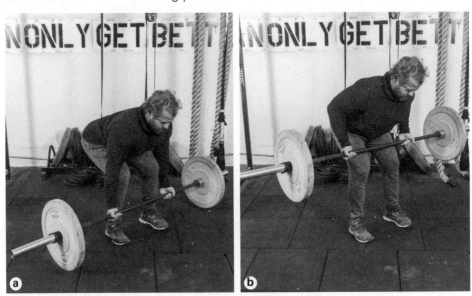

FIGURE 12.15   Reverse-grip row: start *(a)*, and finish *(b)*.

Individuals with long shins or femurs may have trouble keeping the shins vertical without also making the body more vertical. The Yates row may be a good option for these lifters—the body will be at about a 30-degree angle rather than as parallel to the floor as possible, and the weight is rowed to the lower abdominal area (figure 12.16a-b). This will, of course, not train the back muscles in quite the same way that a more traditional position might, but it will allow for a more vertical shin.

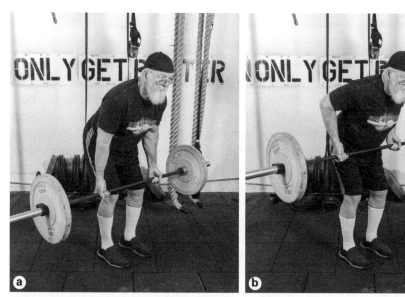

FIGURE 12.16 Yates row: start *(a)*, and finish *(b)*.

Long-legged lifters can also simply use dumbbells or kettlebells for the row so that the shin placement will not get in the way of the lift (figure 12.17*a-b*). Another option for long-legged lifters in particular is to do this exercise on a seated row machine, therefore eliminating the need to worry about leg position. This method will not provide as much specificity to the deadlift position, but it will work the arms and upper back in much the same way as a bent-over reverse-grip deadlift.

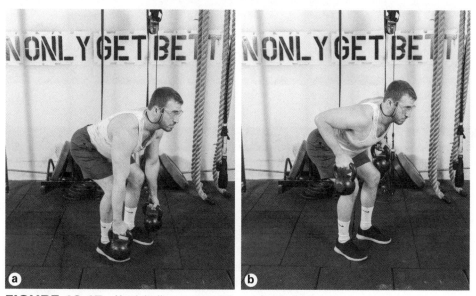

FIGURE 12.17 Kettlebell row: start *(a)*, and finish *(b)*.

Drag Curl

The idea of the barbell drag curl is to remove the stabilizing influence of the deltoids that is normally present in a barbell curl, potentially reducing the risk of shoulder pain that may occur in the standard version of the exercise. Because it removes the influence of the shoulders, the drag curl places more stress on the biceps. The drag curl moves the biceps through a limited range of motion, and it generally requires less weight than a standard biceps curl.

The athlete stands holding a barbell in front of the body, palms supinated as if to curl the bar (figure 12.18a). The athlete pulls their elbows back and drags the barbell up the torso as high as possible (figure 12.18b). The movement is then reversed to return the barbell to the starting position.

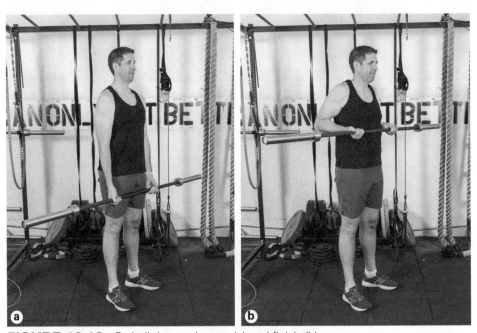

FIGURE 12.18 Barbell drag curl: start *(a)*, and finish *(b)*.

Multiple-Joint Pull Exercises

This section provides a sample of effective multi-joint pull exercises.

Dumbbell Snatch

The dumbbell snatch is a triple extension exercise, and the hips should be the main driver in this movement. This exercise helps build explosive power as well as unilateral overhead strength and stability. Many lifters struggle with the barbell snatch; for these lifters, the dumbbell snatch tends to be easier to learn and to perform. Because most of the momentum in the dumbbell snatch should be coming from the hips, the arm and shoulder are essentially helping to guide the dumbbell in the straightest path overhead.

The dumbbell should be placed on the floor between the feet, under the lifter's center of gravity. Starting in a deadlift position—hips back, shins as perpendicular to the ground as possible, shoulders back, and the curve of the lower back in place—the lifter grasps the dumbbell with a straight arm (figure 12.19a). The lifter then pulls the dumbbell explosively up off the floor, keeping it as close to the body as possible (figure 12.19b). The lifter should keep the arm straight until the hips are fully extended and then quickly shrug the shoulder and pull the elbow up high, as in an upright row, to quickly continue the dumbbell's vertical path. Once the dumbbell is at approximately chest height, the lifter turns the elbow under and continues to guide the dumbbell overhead. When the dumbbell is directly overhead, the lifter then "catches" it by quickly dropping into a squat underneath it; once the dumbbell is stabilized overhead, the lifter stands up to full height, with the abdominals braced, legs locked, and glutes tight (figure 12.19c). Some lifters prefer to do a full squat, and others do a quarter squat. Both of these methods are perfectly acceptable, and the chosen execution will depend on the athlete's goals. One can think of the snatch as a kind of jump—the movement performed by the athlete in the snatch is very similar to a vertical jump.

Long-armed athletes may find this movement to be more challenging, because the dumbbell will have a longer path to travel and may be a bit more of a challenge to stabilize overhead. Some athletes may not have the mobility required to stabilize a weight directly overhead; the dumbbell snatch will not be an ideal exercise for these athletes.

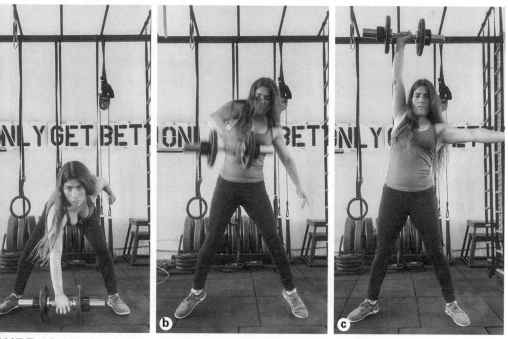

URE 12.19 Dumbbell snatch: start (a), middle (b), and finish position (c).

Lat Pull-Down

The lat pull-down is a good way to target the lats and upper back for those lifters who do not possess the strength to perform classic chin-ups or pull-ups. If band-assisted, eccentric, or even weight-assisted machines aren't an option (or the simple goal is to promote more isolation of the back muscles with less involvement of the core to stabilize the trunk), pull-downs can be a way to do this. Moreover, because this exercise uses less weight than most versions of a pull-up or chin-up, it is easier to customize the motion according to torso angle, tempo, and exact mechanics of the movement. Many lifters use the pull-down to get a handle on starting posture and shoulder control.

Remember what we mentioned in chapter 9 regarding kyphosis and how it can affect a chin-up or pull-up pattern? The fact that the lifter is asked to hang underneath a bar for the start position of either lift can be a problem for those with poor shoulder mobility and limited shoulder flexion due to a kyphotic spine. It is a wise decision to instead use the pull-down pattern since the start and finish position require an angled torso, limiting the degree of shoulder flexion by a few crucial degrees that can keep the shoulder joint in a safer active range of motion (see figure 12.20a-b).

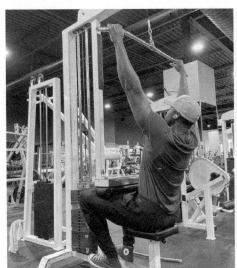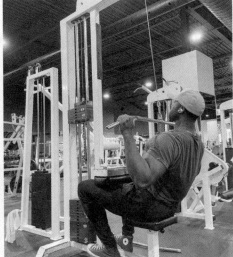

FIGURE 12.20 Lat pull-down: start (a), and finish (b).

The chin-up grip (palms facing in, or supinated) and the pull-up grip (palms facing away, or pronated) are the most common options when holding a standard pull-down bar, but some prefer to substitute the classic V-grip used in many seated row machines (seen in chapter 10). In the end, it's a matter of choice; due to the isolated nature of the movement, it comes down to what the lifter finds provides the best "hit" for the target muscles of the lats and upper back. And there's no harm in cycling among various grips.

Considerations for Lower Body Training

The lower body is a slightly different animal when it comes to accessory work. Many options for lower body exercises involve movements that are compound in nature, which can rival the amount of energy expenditure required for a squat or deadlift exercise. For those reasons, accessory work on leg day or other workouts involving such patterns should be considered carefully. As a whole, many accessory movements for the lower body often favor one side of the leg—quadriceps- and hip flexor–based exercises and hamstring- and glute-based exercises. The calves and adductor group (typically considered the two missing pieces from this list) are involved as tertiary muscle groups in most of the lifts under each category; however, accessory movements that target these muscles directly are also important and worth including in this section. But first, it's time to expose one unicorn exercise that deserves more attention than it receives.

Leg Press

With all things equal, the leg press exercise is a terrific supplement to lower body lifts, for the principal reason that it involves a co-contraction of most of the muscles of the lower body (thanks to simultaneous knee and hip flexion), and it also allows for plenty of loading for a challenging stimulus. There are different setups for the leg press machine—some are positioned horizontally where the lifter sits nearly upright in the seat and presses the platform straight out (figure 12.21a), whereas others are positioned with more of a vertical orientation, where the lifter presses the platform from their seated position at ground level, away from the floor at a 45-degree angle (figure 12.21b).

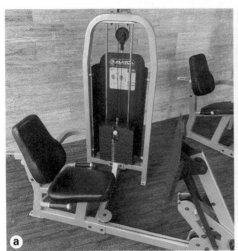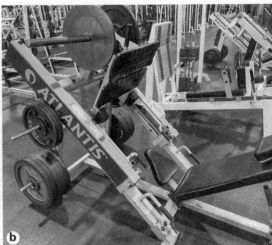

FIGURE 12.21   Horizontal orientation on the leg press machine *(a)*, and 45-degree orientation

Another thing that makes the leg press unique is that it's a compound, bilateral-stance lower body exercise that completely immobilizes the torso. Done properly, the torso angle doesn't change through the duration of the movement, and stress forces on the spine are reduced compared with a squat pattern because the "floor" moves toward and away from the lifter, rather than the lifter moving toward and away from the floor.

Adjusting the foot position on the leg press machine is what makes it an exercise that can bias one group of muscles over another. Depending on a lifter's leverages and mechanics, the quadriceps can be activated much more (e.g., using a lower, narrower foot position on the platform), or the gluteal muscles can be activated with a higher, wider foot position (Da Silva et al. 2008). These adjustments can work well for a longer-legged lifter who experiences knee stress during certain foot stances or an uncomfortable hip position. A lifter who has shorter legs or a more compact frame may struggle to emphasize dorsiflexion or quadriceps activity, so a foot position lower on the platform can help work these ranges of motion.

Because of the limited range of motion for hip extension, the emphasis in any leg press will be deep hip and knee flexion. There's little to be gained by performing this movement with a partial range of motion; the leg is already limited in its extension range because the body is prevented from becoming completely straightened. It should be a lifter's goal to move through the full range of motion, as long as the hips remain squared on the seat and the spine does not round. Like any exercise, approaching the movement maturely by considering rep quality before adding weight is smart.

The leg press can also use gravity to increase range of motion at the ankle joint. Many lifters of varying body types (especially lifters with tall bodies or long legs) would functionally benefit from improved dorsiflexion, but when standing and bearing their own weight, it's too challenging to get into deep ranges of dorsiflexion with the foot planted on the ground. When inverted and set up on a low-foot-position leg press, it's easier to make the knees pass forward over the toes while the heel remains planted on the platform. This should be used to a lifter's advantage if it's a specific area of difficulty.

Walking Lunge

Lunges are a go-to supplementary exercise that also involve a co-contraction of all major muscles of the leg. However, like the leg press, changes to the mechanics and geometry of the lift can allow a lifter to favor certain muscles over others.

First, it's important to explain why we've chosen a walking lunge and not a stationary lunge as our preferred version. In the case of a forward stationary lunge, there needs to be a directional change on each completed repetition. This means the leading leg needs to stop the forward momentum of the body and then push off against the ground using the foot (along with the quads and connective tissue of the knee) in order to return to the starting position. As the weight increases in this exercise, it begins to transcend the muscular strength of the lifter and start interfering with the ease of accomplishing the task. Simply put, it becomes cumbersome to do this with heavier loads; breaking kinetic energy is a big ask for the joints, and we've found it leads to a faster technical breakdown compared with a walking lunge.

In the case of the walking lunge, the body is more free to continue its forward motion, for a smooth and solid foot strike and an unbroken hip extension—another huge benefit not mentioned earlier.

In both cases, properly lunging means ensuring sufficient alignment of the knee, hip, and shoulder joints on each side. It's a very common tendency for a lifter's knees to fall in toward the midline when faced with a unilateral exercise (like this one). This usually leads to a drop in one hip, creating misalignment throughout the body and spelling danger for load-bearing joints. There are many reasons why this knee collapse happens. Rather than list them all, it's more sensible to provide this checklist for your athletes to consider when performing the lunge:

- On each stride, the foot should be firmly planted on the ground from toe to heel, and the arch in the foot must be maintained.
- The knees should point where the toes face, and not toward a point narrower than this stance.
- If holding dumbbells, it's ideal to stop them from swinging to maintain balance. That will mean bracing the upper body. Attempting to flex the triceps for the duration of the set can be very helpful because it forces the arms to remain straight and fixed.

Respecting these rules can take technical flaws out of the picture when explaining knee collapse, leaving a lifter in a better place to examine specific muscular weaknesses as culprits. The glutes and inner thighs, respectively, can act as large knee stabilizers in unilateral exercises, and their weakness—especially compared with one another—can influence the tracking of the knee joint. During bilateral-stance exercises, this issue is slightly easier to hide since the base of support is wider.

Biasing the lunge to target more of the quads and hips or more of the glutes and hamstrings is as simple as keeping the heel planted and choosing the stride length that suits the goals of the lifter. For a quad and hip emphasis, using a shorter stride and keeping the torso vertical means the knee of the leading leg will need to travel far over the toe (and enter deep flexion) in order for the knee of the trailing leg to make it to or near the floor (figure 12.24a). In other words, for the back knee to touch the ground with a close-

A Quick Note: Women and Walking Lunges

Women would do well to pay special attention to this portion of their lunge mechanics, because the majority of women possess what's known as the Q angle (figure 12.22). Compared with the male anatomy, the female anatomy tends to have wider hips relative to the rest of the body. As such, women's femurs have a more distinct slanted pattern than do men's.

Because of this difference in anatomy, it's much easier for knee valgus (medial translation of the knee) to occur since the anatomy already puts a woman's body halfway there without trying. On that note, the recommendation for lunge variations would be

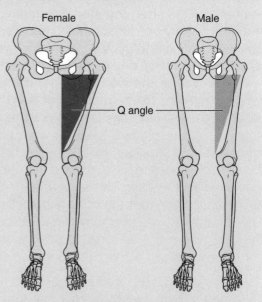

Figure 12.22   Female (left) and male (right) versions of the lower skeleton with Q angle from hip to knee highlighted.

to step slightly wider—nothing tremendously noticeable; a few inches wider is perfectly fine—in order to counter valgus. This position will place the foot under the hip socket and allow the knee to correspond to this alignment.

stance lunge, the torso will need to remain vertical. A close stride and a deep knee-over-toe position will mean more work for the knee extensors—the quadriceps group—on each stride. Entering a slight posterior pelvic tilt while performing lunges in this fashion can further benefit the quads' involvement because this change in pelvic position reduces the tension placed on the hamstring group. Because the hamstrings originate on the ischial tuberosity of the pelvis (figure 12.23), posteriorly tilting the pelvis (to bring the spine into mild flexion) can decrease the distance between the origin and insertion point of the hamstrings, making for a less taut muscle group that won't contribute to the pattern as readily.

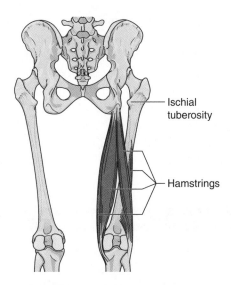

FIGURE 12.23 Hamstrings muscles, highlighting attachment point to ischial tuberosity.

Conversely, to favor the glutes and hamstrings, the angle in question needs to shift from the knee joint to the hip joint. Therefore, decreasing the degree of flexion at the knee and increasing the degree of flexion at the hip will result in a greater emphasis on the hip extensors—primarily the glutes and hamstrings (figure 12.24b). In practice, that would translate to a slightly longer stride, with a distinct forward lean at the torso, while maintaining a

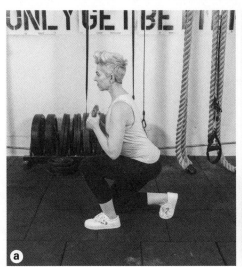
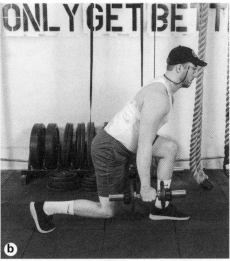

FIGURE 12.24 Bottom lunge position: quad and hip emphasis (a), and glute and hamstring emphasis (b).

neutral or slightly arched lumbar spine to distance the ischial tuberosity from the knee on the working leg, thus making the hamstrings taut. With a more vertical front shin, the lunge pattern can function similar to that of a box squat in forcing the posterior chain to be slightly more active than otherwise.

The walking lunge can double as a very draining conditioning exercise, and higher reps are recommended. Remember: The quadriceps—which will indeed be involved regardless of the variation performed—tend to respond well to muscular endurance work, so this exercise presents an opportunity to exploit that element of fitness. Sets of at least 20 walking strides should be aimed for.

Single-Leg Deadlift

The single-leg deadlift can be an excellent way to train the strength and stability of each leg and to improve an athlete's balance and coordination throughout a range of motion. It also enhances the strength and stability of the muscles of the torso. The single-leg deadlift has a number of variations that can be selected based on the abilities of the athlete. Any of these movements can be performed by holding a barbell, dumbbell, or kettlebell in each hand, or they can be done unilaterally, with a dumbbell or kettlebell in one hand only.

The one-arm and one-leg version of this exercise will generally challenge the lifter's balance the most and will also serve as an anti-rotation exercise. It is recommended that the loaded arm and the standing leg be on the same side of the body.

For each of the following variations, the following standard cues will be used:

- "Spine rigid/slightly arched"
- "Movement occurs at the hip only"
- "Shoulders level with each other"
- "Hips level with each other"
- "The working leg is unlocked, not overly bent"
- "Stop hinging before the back starts to round—the weights do not need to touch the floor"

For many people, achieving balance with any version of the single-leg deadlift can be a challenge. One useful cue is to tell the lifter to keep the eyes fixed on an object or spot on the ground a few feet in front of them for the duration of the movement. Moving the eyes around can make balancing on one leg much more challenging.

Staggered-Stance Single-Leg Deadlift

This variation of the single-leg deadlift is best for athletes who have difficulty performing a single-leg deadlift without assistance. In this exercise, the athlete places one foot slightly behind the other. The toe of the back leg remains on the ground for balance purposes only—the bulk of the weight will remain on the front leg. Keeping the knee of the loaded leg unlocked, the athlete keeps the spine rigid and hinges at the loaded hip, following all the standard cues, and then returns to the starting position (figure 12.25a).

Bent-Leg Single-Leg Deadlift

In this version, the free leg remains slightly bent and stays off the ground while the lifter performs the single-leg deadlift according to the standard cues (figure 12.25b). In this variation, the back lever is shorter and therefore easier to control for the duration of the exercise.

Straight-Leg Single-Leg Deadlift

The most challenging of the variations listed here, the straight-leg single-leg deadlift (figure 12.25c) requires the athlete to keep the free leg locked and in line with the rest of the body, much like a seesaw. The athlete moves the body and the leg as one unit, so if the torso is moving, the free leg is also moving with it at the same pace. In this version, the athlete's range of motion may be more limited because it may be more of a challenge to maintain the integrity of the spine through the same range of motion as the other versions of this exercise.

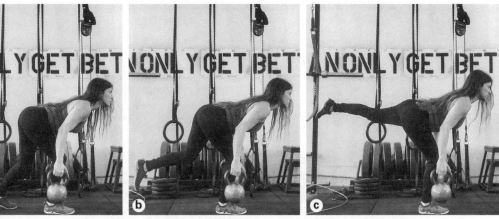

GURE 12.25   Staggered-stance single-leg deadlift (a), bent-leg single-leg deadlift (b), and ʃight-leg single-leg deadlift (c).

Eccentric Nordic Curl (Target: Posterior Chain)

The typical Nordic curl requires a lifter to kneel, secure the heels under an immovable object, and, using body-weight strength, fall forward (figure 12.26a) to as far a range of motion as possible (the floor being the maximum range available). The body shouldn't fold much at the hip joint—a fixed joint angle of 10 to 15 degrees of flexion is allowable throughout the duration of the movement. Once the bottom is reached (figure 12.26b), the next step is to return to the start position, using the same form—primarily relying on the hamstrings to do so. The issue that arises is simple: Most people aren't strong enough to perform these cleanly. Even strong lifters can struggle with the movement if they don't have a body size conducive to excellent

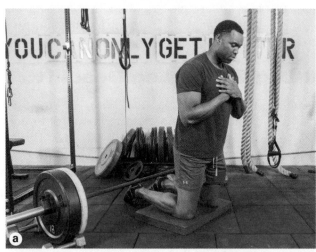

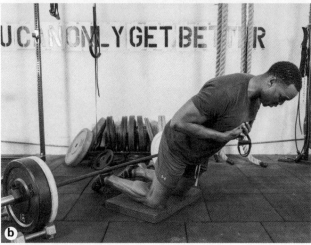

FIGURE 12.26   Nordic curl: start (a), and finish (b).

performance in the lift (it's a big ask to get a 6-foot-6, 270-pound individual to ace a set of Nordic curls). Attention can start shifting away from the hamstrings and into more sensitive areas like the ligaments of the knee, lumbar spine, and hamstring tendon attachments—which distracts a lifter from the movement's benefits.

For that reason, focusing on the eccentric portion of the movement only can be a saving grace that keeps the attention on the correct areas. Aiming to descend all the way to the floor while "braking" as much as possible makes the hamstring group work eccentrically, exploiting the limits of their strength. A lifter should aim to make the descent last between 5 and 10 seconds, then support themselves on the floor using the hands once reached. A brisk push-up motion to get back to the top position is recommended because no concentric activity should be involved. Since there is no change of direction to place additional demand on the connective tissue, the lifter can focus on complete muscular deceleration strength of the hamstrings. Such deceleration strength is a vital attribute in other training movements like the deadlift and squat, as well as locomotive movements like efficient sprinting (in addition to hip extension to push off the ground, the hamstrings play a vital role in decelerating the shin of the leading leg on each stride, in order not to reach out and overstride). During a set, it can be expected that as the lifter fatigues, they will not be able to control the descent as well as at the start, so reps should be kept under 10 to ensure quality.

Nordic Curl Hip Hinge

As great as the eccentric Nordic curl is—increased safety for joints and more overall accessibility when compared with the full Nordic curl—a number of clients we have worked with have experienced discomfort from these variations in the form of ligament stress in the knee. There is no research on this subject, but here is our philosophy. The same way a leg extension can be unfriendly to the knees of certain clients because of anterior shear (this phenomenon happens during leg extensions since they are an open chain movement, and the tibia is moving while the femur is held fixed when seated in position), we believe that in the case of the Nordic curl, the femur is now moving while the tibia is held fixed, meaning the same phenomenon is happening in the form of *posterior* shear. As the weight of a lifter's upper body begins to fall forward, this joint stress can make itself manifest. Immobilizing the femur while sharing the responsibility of the hamstrings' action is a way to improve the situation.

Whereas Nordic curls focus very dominantly on knee extension and flexion, the Nordic curl hip hinge (figure 12.27a-b) differs even from the eccentric variation. The femur is kept in one place, so the knee joint endures fewer

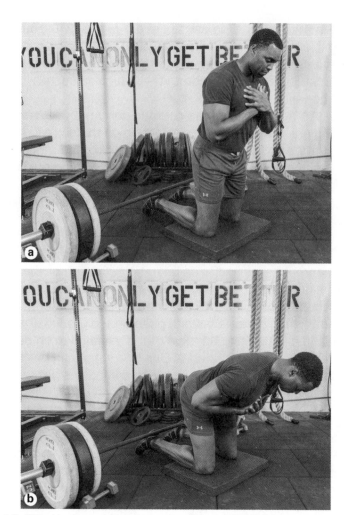

FIGURE 12.27   Nordic curl hip hinge: start *(a)*, and finish *(b)*.

stress forces than would be encountered from a constant change in load-bearing angle. Here, the hamstrings are asked to simultaneously hold an isometric knee flexion and actively extend the hip joint, making for a much more complete engagement that's friendlier to the joints. Adding a mild load while being honest with the reps will prove that it doesn't take much to really torch the hamstrings.

This movement can be done for slightly higher rep ranges than the eccentric Nordic curl, considering the focus is less on deceleration, or negative reps. Focusing on sets of 12 to 15 repetitions is perfectly acceptable here.

Reverse Nordic Curl (Target: Anterior Chain)

Very few exercises target the quads from a fully lengthened position. Most exercises call for knee extension while the hip is also flexed. Seated leg extensions, squats, and lunges are all examples of this. The reverse Nordic curl allows the hip to start and remain in extension through the duration of each repetition, which can build strength exclusively in knee extension by taking advantage of the length–tension relationship (emphasizing the amount of tension the quads can create as a feature of their length). There are four quadriceps muscles, and this may be a way to better target harder-to-isolate quads like the vastus intermedius and rectus femoris.

To perform this exercise, a lifter assumes a hip-width, tall kneeling position on a mat with the insteps facing down (figure 12.28a) (shoelaces on the mat). Maintaining an erect body, the lifter leans back toward the floor, pressing hard into the ground with the feet and shins in order to create tension through the quads, thus braking the descent (figure 12.28b). It's important to keep the glutes contracted the entire time to avoid overarching the lower back. This will also ensure the abdominals are remaining engaged, which is crucial for overall tension and bracing. The eccentric phase of the lift should stop when the lifter feels at the border between ease of completion and technical failure, and then the concentric portion of the movement begins, following all the same cues to return to an upright position. The hands can be crossed over the chest—a typical default for most lifters seeking a comfortable hand position. Some lifters keep the arms extended in front of them for a better sense of balance. To progress this exercise, hugging a light weight plate in front of the body—only when maximal range of motion has been achieved with body weight—is recommended. Many conditioned, shorter lifters will find making this adjustment fitting.

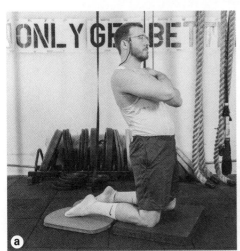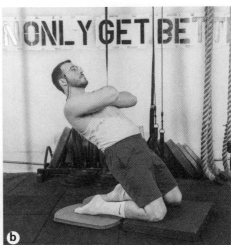

FIGURE 12.28   Reverse Nordic curl: start *(a)*, and finish *(b)*.

Band-Assisted Reverse Nordics: Tall; Big All Over

Bigger, heavier lifters and those who have longer levers will have greater loading on the quads and knees for this exercise compared with lifters with compact frames. A combination of a higher body weight and longer lever arms means a great deal of variation in the amount of force placed on the fulcrum (the knee), as it would be for any lever. A band wrapped above forehead level on a post or sturdy object can take some of the lifter's body weight, allowing for a suitable range of motion that isn't limited by knee health or quad strength (figure 12.29a and 12.29b). Holding the band with both hands outstretched in front of the body as a guide will encourage proper form and help the lifter out of the bottom position to exit deep knee flexion. As the lifter improves in strength, body composition, or both, the thickness of the band can be reduced, until no band is needed.

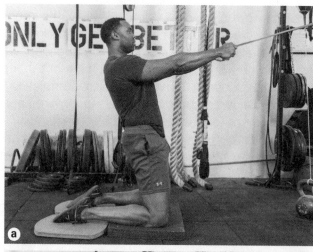

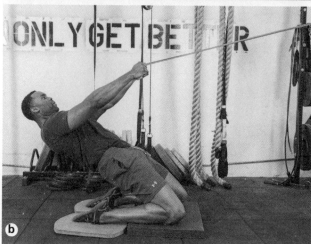

FIGURE 12.29   Band-assisted reverse Nordic curl: start *(a)*, and finish *(b)*.

Reverse Hyperextensions

Reverse hyperextensions can be performed on a bench, on a hyperextension bench (figure 12.30*a-b*), or on a reverse hyperextension machine. A reverse hyperextension machine will provide the best range of motion and loading capacity of these three options, but any of the three variations will provide good benefits. Reverse hyperextensions can be an excellent way to build strength in the lower back, glutes, and hamstrings while keeping the spine supported.

In this exercise, the athlete lies facedown on whichever apparatus they are using, with their legs off the edge of the bench or machine and the hip joints at the edge of the machine or bench so that they can move freely at the hips. Starting with the legs in the lowest position possible, the athlete raises the legs, keeping them straight and under control, up to a horizontal position. The athlete holds the top position for about one second by contracting the glutes and keeping the legs straight and then lowers the legs under control back to the starting position. An athlete with shorter femurs performing this exercise on a bench might be able to bring the knees all the way in at the bottom of the exercise so that the thighs are perpendicular to the floor and the shins are parallel to the floor. When initiating the movement, the athlete simply straightens the legs behind them and raises the legs to

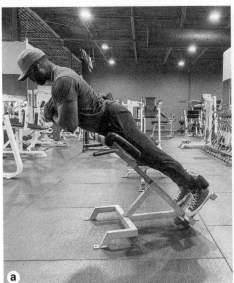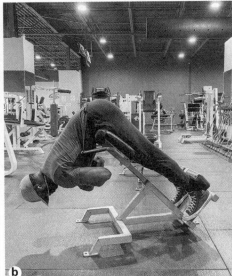

FIGURE 12.30 Reverse bench hyperextension: start *(a)*, and finish *(b)*.

parallel to the floor. To load this exercise when performing it on a bench or hyperextension bench, the athlete can use ankle weights, hold a dumbbell between the feet, or attach a weight to a rope that is hung around the ankles.

The reverse hyperextension provides the hamstring- and glute-strengthening benefits of movements such as hip thrusts, good mornings, traditional back extensions, and Romanian deadlifts without putting excess strain on the spine or taxing the grip. It can be a more challenging exercise for long-legged lifters because the load will be further from the fulcrum (i.e., the hips) than in a short-legged athlete. This may simply translate to using a lighter load for long-legged athletes. Reverse hyperextensions might be uncomfortable for athletes who are big all over and have more mass around the midsection. Performing this movement on a glute-ham raise apparatus might solve this issue, because the athlete can arrange the pads so that the midsection is not compressed by anything.

Rear-Foot-Elevated Split Squat

It's sensible to start by explaining the distinction between a split squat and a lunge, because they often get mistaken for one another. A lunge involves movement and starts with both feet together in a bilateral standing position. The lifter steps forward (or backward) into a split stance and then returns to the starting position either by pushing back or by driving through to the next stride, like the walking lunges mentioned earlier. In short, the lunge is a dynamic movement. Split squat variations, however, are stationary in nature. The feet begin and end in a split stance, not a bilateral one. To take things a step further, the general orientation of the split squat movement is up and down. Since there is no forward momentum and all the reps are performed on one side before switching legs, the back knee can be a greater area of focus to drop straight downward for a more upright torso. In the case of the lunge pattern, there tends to be more coaching toward an allowance for a slightly forward momentum during the lift's execution; doing so can benefit the transition from one leg to the other.

Taking a split squat to a different degree by elevating the rear foot on a bench or pad simultaneously stimulates the lower body musculature of the leading leg while placing the hip and quadriceps groups of the trailing leg in a deep loaded stretch. For lifters who struggle with depth and range of motion in the squat because of hip immobility, this exercise can be a worthy supplement to their programming.

Like lunges, the area of emphasis can be slightly different depending on the stance assumed. Using a shorter stride distance and maintaining heel contact on the front leg will make the quads work more than a longer stance and leaning forward slightly at the hip (which will emphasize more of the hamstrings and glutes).

There are two common foot positions when setting up the rear-foot-elevated split squat. In both cases, the front foot is planted squarely on the ground. The rear foot is placed on the bench with either the toe down (known as "squishing the bug") (figure 12.31a) or the instep down so the shoelaces are against the surface of the bench or pad instead (figure 12.31b). Each is permissible, but each presents mild disadvantages, depending on the population doing them.

In the case of squishing the bug, it's a lot to ask of the construction of the foot since the deeper the trailing leg travels, the more the trailing foot needs to enter plantar flexion in order to maintain contact with the bench. We've seen more than a few cases where the lifter complains of stress between the metatarsal joints of the feet when performing the exercise in this way. To remain comfortable when assuming this setup, most lifters will cut their range of motion by finishing each rep in a shallower-than-ideal position, which can defeat one of the purposes of the exercise.

Alternatively, the shoelaces-down approach may be more accessible for lifters and solves the problems of ligament stress in the foot and insufficient depth. However, if the lifter in question has issues with pointing the toes or getting into deep plantar flexion by way of a stretch, they'll have trouble

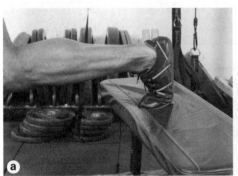
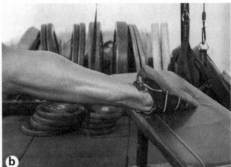
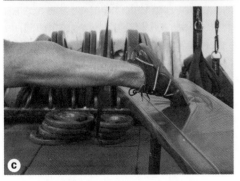

FIGURE 12.31 Rear-foot-elevated split squat: "squish the bug" foot position (a), shoelaces down (b), and foot position for tall lifters (c).

getting their full instep flush with the bench. Also, the bench height may be too low for tall lifters to get into this position when standing. As a result, at the end of each rep, the shoelaces leave the bench or pad, such that only the tip of the toe is left in contact with it (figure 12.31c), causing balance issues.

The solution to these problems is to find a surface that naturally allows the foot to hook itself around the edge of the apparatus for a more comfortable ascent and descent that's not truncated by the confines of ankle mobility, height, or flexibility. Some companies make equipment with the sole purpose of split squatting; such an apparatus has a round, padded base point that is adjustable in height for the foot to be placed on. However, if this isn't available, it's possible to replicate this setup using a Smith machine and bar pad. Finally, using the head of an inclined bench creates an angle that wedges perfectly into the instep, allowing the foot to hook onto the bench for a split squat that's free of wavering or shallow ranges.

Our recommendation for the rear-foot-elevated split squat is sets of 8 to 12 reps per leg in order to focus on patterning, mobility benefits, and muscular endurance of the quads and glutes. However, many lifters also use the movement for single-leg strength training, lifting heavier dumbbells or a heavier barbell (back or front loaded) for lower reps—typically 4 to 6 reps per leg. In each case, this exercise provides value.

Short Lifters: Rear-Foot-Elevated Split Squat With Deficit

Lifters with shorter legs can face the direct opposite problem outlined in the previous section. Whereas taller lifters will have the problem of a low bench obstructing their range of motion at the ankle, shorter lifters may find that a high bench height obstructs the depth they can achieve at the knee and hip of the trailing leg. Since the foot is very elevated for their frame and size, an aggressive hip and quad stretch is needed to make the knee touch the floor, which might not be in the realm of possibility for the lifter. Adding a raised surface (a few inches) for the front foot can help balance the scales by changing the elevation of the rear foot (figure 12.32a). In addition, this serves a second purpose by creating a deficit; the trailing knee is now able to travel below the level of the front foot, which can be the answer to plenty of frustrations shorter lifters will have due to insufficient ranges of motion (figure 12.32b).

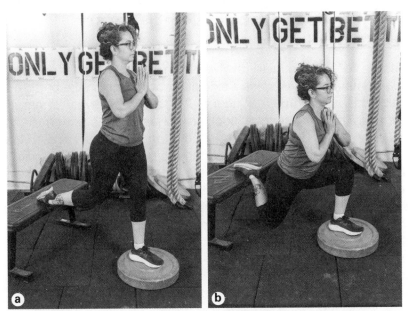

FIGURE 12.32   Deficit rear-foot-elevated split squat: start *(a)*, and finish *(b)*.

Copenhagen Plank

The adductor group can be a very weak link that many lifters overlook in the name of bilateral-stance exercises. Their weakness and lack of specific training can be a contributing factor to knee collapse (known as valgus) when performing unilateral or bilateral work. A multitude of exercises focus on the inner thigh, but few actually train the inner thighs to bear load while the body is tall, meaning when the hips are extended.

Think about a seated abduction/adduction machine found at most commercial gyms: The body isn't bearing much load while performing the pattern in any place other than the inner thigh, from a poor force angle at that. It's not realistic to think this variation of the movement will translate much to squat, deadlift, or lunge performance because of the orientation of the movement.

Instead, using a bench for a Copenhagen plank can be a better way to seek alignment at the hip and knee joint, while bearing load in a much more practical way. A number of Copenhagen plank variations can benefit a lifter, and it makes sense to go over our top choices.

Straight Leg: Short; Long Torso and Short Legs

Setting up for this exercise involves lying on the floor perpendicular to a standard flat bench. Assuming a side plank by resting on the bottom forearm and elbow is recommended (figure 12.33a). Alternatively, lifters can prop up the supporting arm with a block or low platform as preferred. Next, the lifter places the inside (medial side) of the top foot and ankle onto the bench and presses hard through that foot into the bench in order to raise the hips off the ground. The lifter then raises the bottom leg by keeping a straight knee and squeezing up to bench level (figure 12.33b). The lifter performs these squeezes for slow and controlled reps, focusing on the engagement of the adductors in both legs in order to close the distance between the thighs and feet.

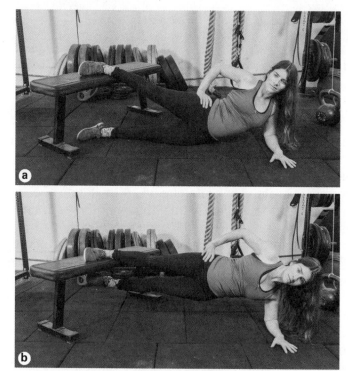

FIGURE 12.33   Straight-legged Copenhagen plank: start *(a)*, and finish *(b)*.

This is a recommended variation for lifters who have shorter extremities or who are smaller and lighter overall. A larger lever arm or a heavier body-weight load will produce greater stress forces on the medial knee as the joint bearing the majority of the lifter's weight, and this can result in pain or discomfort that distracts the lifter from the benefits of the movement for the adductors.

Bent Knee: Big All Over; Long Legs

Big lifters can solve the problem just mentioned by shortening the lever arm. Placing the full shin on the bench allows the lifter's adductors to deal with a more manageable load relative to the body weight; this also spares the knee joint of any stress on the medial side. Since the knee is now banked on the bench as well, its safety is a given, which is a crucial adjustment to a Copenhagen plank in its basic form (figure 12.34a). To accommodate for the change in levers, the bottom leg can also switch from being straight to being in a runner's pose, with the hip and knee flexed to 90-degree angles (figure 12.34b). The lifter's goal should be to make the bottom hip and thigh contact the floor on each rep. (Of course, for a full range of motion, a concentric pattern brings the body up to the height of the bench.)

Because this is a body-weight exercise, focusing on sets of 10 or more reps per side is reasonable. Most lifters find this pattern more worthwhile when making the aim muscular endurance rather than top-end strength. Slow and controlled lifting tempos allow a lifter to focus on the target muscles.

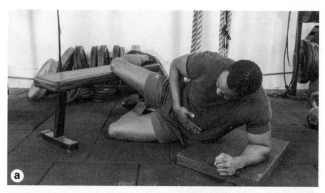

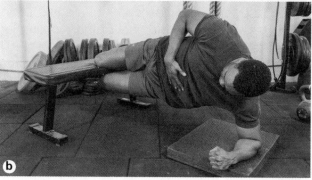

FIGURE 12.34   Bent-legged Copenhagen plank: start *(a),* and finish *(b).*

Copenhagen Plank: Isotonic Versus Isometric

Lastly, a lifter has the option of performing Copenhagen planks in an isotonic fashion (using concentric or eccentric reps) or an isometric fashion (using a strict hold, as in a typical plank). Either is acceptable depending on what the lifter prefers for a given workout. However, lifters dealing with lower body injury or who are lacking strength in the exercise itself may benefit from opting for isometric holds to reduce the risk of further injury.

Cossack Squat

Like the Copenhagen plank, the Cossack squat is a movement that does something unique: It trains the legs outside of the sagittal plane. This lateral movement is vital for total joint health and the development of athleticism, which is why we include it as an essential assistance exercise. The Cossack squat is very dependent on mobility and single-leg strength, and it's no surprise that many lifters find it challenging, despite having good performance by the numbers in exercises like squats or deadlifts.

Since the body is shifting laterally and medially (not forward and backward or up and down), the lifter has to adjust to a different form of movement and a plane of force and deceleration they may not be used to. Depending on body type, special considerations may need to be made. But first, let's go over the basics of the pattern's execution.

The lifter sets the feet in a wide sumo stance, with the toes pointing outward (figure 12.35a). Next, they shift their body weight over one foot as the other leg straightens at the knee. It's okay for the toe to leave the floor and point up toward the roof while this happens. As the lifter shifts their body weight over one leg, they begin to descend into a squat position on that leg (figure 12.35b). This will require the heel of the working leg to remain planted and the torso to be positioned squarely over the thigh. The lifter will maintain a tall posture and return to the start position before repeating on

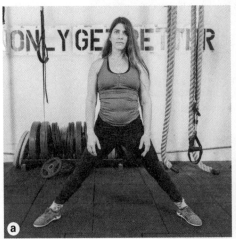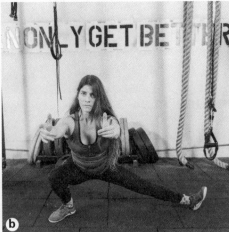

FIGURE 12.35 Cossack squat: start (a), and finish (b).

the same side or alternating legs. The emphasis should be on maintaining tension throughout the duration of the lift, even though the aim is for full range of motion on either side.

Counterbalance: Long Legs and Short Torso

Certain body types will have difficulty with this movement in its basic form; it's an exercise that's much friendlier to trainees with longer torsos and shorter legs. A lifter with longer legs and a shorter torso will inevitably have trouble staying upright and have a tendency to fall backward owing to a lack of counterbalance. Even if dorsiflexion health is strong, emphasizing a single leg while traveling laterally can frustrate the ability to remain vertical when support isn't present. For that reason, holding a single dumbbell or kettlebell with outstretched arms can give the lifter a countering load to sit against; similar to a front-loaded squat pattern, this can encourage a more vertical torso and better balance.

Box Cossack Squat: Big All Over; Tall

Traveling a great distance downward can be a big ask for a lifter doing a normal squat, as you've learned. Adding a Cossack squat into the mix can compound those frustrations, and for that reason, including a target is in good order (figure 12.36a). Like tall people, big and heavy lifters can also benefit from making this adjustment to reduce risk of single-leg load bearing in such a technical movement. Cutting away some of the available range of motion by setting up a step with removable risers is a smart way to build up to a healthy and strong full range of motion when the time comes for it (figure 12.36b).

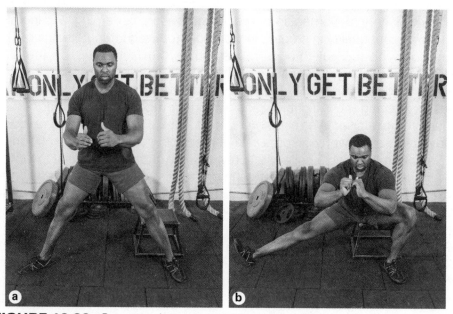

FIGURE 12.36   Box cossack squat: start (a), and finish (b).

Barbell Hip Thrust

Hip thrust variations can be a powerful addition to a lower body training program, primarily because they allow the body to perform a loaded hip extension without the angle of force imposed by a deadlift or squat. Even though the hinge pattern is still being used, having the weight positioned across the hips (rather than on the shoulders or floor) allows the glutes to be recruited through a much greater percentage of the active range of motion. Also, in comparison to squats, there is less quad involvement to distract from the activity of the hip extensors.

To set up the barbell hip thrust, the lifter sits on the floor with the upper back placed against the long edge of a stable bench or other surface. The bar is placed across the hips. (We've found that it is generally more comfortable to use a bar pad to soften the points of contact between bar and body, especially when lifting heavier loads.) Keeping a hip-width foot base with approximately 90-degree angles at the knees, and keeping the heels flat on the floor, the lifter uses the glutes to drive the hips to full extension, using the bench as a pivot point for the upper back.

It's worth noting that lifters with longer legs and shorter torsos will have a harder time finding the ideal back position on a standard bench, because the bench will contact a higher point on their backs and may obstruct their arms. In such a case, using the end edge of a bench may be a suitable option.

Cable Pull-Through

Similar to the hip thrust, the pull-through creates a different angle of force from which hip extension can be trained. Whereas the hip thrust can be loaded appreciably for true training purposes and progressive overload, the pull-through cannot quite be approached the same way. It is better viewed as an accessory movement in the vein of activation, patterning, and ingraining movement quality in preparation for more focused strength training. The limitation with the pull-through movement is the fact that once the load becomes too heavy, it becomes a difficult task to simply maintain balance without getting pulled backward by the forces of the cable and load. For that reason, keeping the weight low and aiming for more reps is a smarter way to use the exercise. We recommend it be done at the beginning of lower body or hip-dominant workouts as a primer to ingrain technical proficiency.

Setting up at a cable pulley station with a low attachment point (near the shins works best), use a rope attachment to allow the lifter to straddle the pulley while facing away from it (figure 12.37a). The aim is to achieve a torso position parallel to the floor using a neutral spine, with the arms kept long and minimally involved as anything more than anchors to the load (figure 12.37b). Done properly, this will create the same geometry as a deadlift, although the angle of force will be similar to a hip thrust. As such, it will be easier to contract the glutes and hamstrings through the entire range of

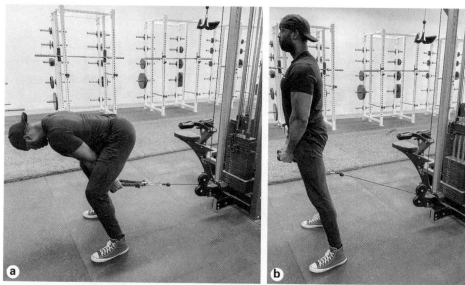

FIGURE 12.37   Cable pull-through: start *(a)*, and finish *(b)*.

motion, and there will be less opportunity for loading stress to be shifted away from the target muscles.

For lifters who don't have access to a cable pulley machine, attaching a band of desired thickness to any stable post will suffice.

Leg Extensions and Leg Curls

Leg extensions and leg curls are often thought of as a pair, simply because they're single-joint isolation machine exercises that zero in on the thigh (the front of the thigh with leg extensions and the back of the thigh with leg curls). There aren't too many cues to follow to perform either movement correctly; in other words, it's pretty hard to mess up these exercises. However, optimizing the movements depends on the fine details of the setup; it has more to do with the machine and less to do with the individual.

Leg Extensions

The general guideline for performing seated leg extensions is that the seat position should be adjusted to place the lifter in a spot where the knees are aligned with the axis of the machine (figure 12.38*a-b*). This can be done by moving the back support of the seat forward or backward, depending on preference and anthropometry. Similarly, most leg extension machines also have an adjustable shin pad that can move upward or downward depending on leg length. For a larger lever arm, placing the pad closer to the ankle would be desired. This placement will increase the focus on the quads, but it's important to note that it will also create more knee stress.

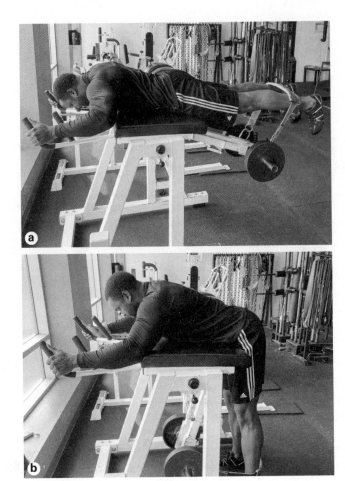

FIGURE 12.38   Leg extension: start *(a)*, and finish *(b)*.

Leg Curls

The prone leg curl focuses on the hamstrings as a knee flexor, not a hip extensor. This makes it a unique exercise to use to properly supplement a strength training program. As with leg extensions, the position of the shin pad can be adjusted, and the greater lever arm for the hamstrings results from the pad being closer to the heel when lying prone. The legs should be near (but not at) full extension in the starting position, with a little bit of room for the weight stack to return to the resting position (figure 12.39*a-b*). This is an important distinction to make: This differs from keeping the legs completely extended under tension. Since this movement involves very few synergists, almost all of the patterning is focused around the knee joint. Beginning each rep at 5 degrees of knee flexion rather than a full knee extension reduces the risk of loaded hyperextension of the knee, which would result in unwanted tendon or ligament stress.

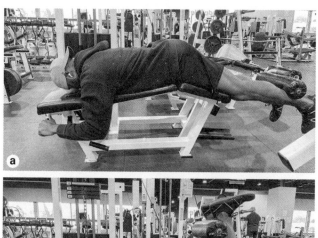

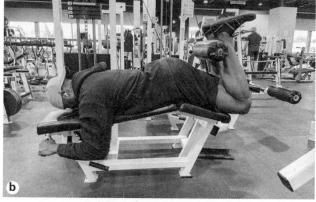

FIGURE 12.39 Leg curl: start *(a)*, and finish *(b)*.

For both exercises, customizing the leg and foot width and angle can be used for emphasizing certain parts of each target muscle group. However, the square hip-width stance is most recommended, with a fairly neutral foot angle (not fully dorsiflexed, nor fully plantar-flexed).

Accessory work can be just as important as the big stuff. It's important to remember that squats, deadlifts, chin-ups, rows, and presses are all sagittal plane movements. Training them can improve a lifter's strength, muscularity, and even athleticism on a basic level, but they're still missing frontal and transverse plane work that can help make gains complete. As a bonus, accessory movements serve the bigger lifts by adding training volume to weak links, stabilizing muscles, and working muscles that aren't often isolated (but rather act as synergists to other groups during those big lifts). The result can be significant improvements in performance. The moral of the story: Programming accessory work is worth its weight in gold.

Chapter 13

Considerations for Conditioning Training

Although this book is predominantly geared toward strength development and resistance training, it's fitting to include a category dedicated to conditioning work. We are believers in well-rounded fitness, and as explained in our opening chapters, a proper sense of balance needs to be applied to weight training—especially as a lifter exits their "juvenile years" as a trainee, and as a human being. Training for numerical performance year round is something a young adult can have no problem with, but it doesn't account for other lifters who may be older, who may have been training for decades, or who have prior injuries to care for amid responsibilities of life.

Training to sustain strength and improve fitness and overall health should be viewed very differently by the 40- or 50-year-old who's already got a foundation than by a 21-year-old who's never touched a barbell a day in their life. Regardless of the starting point, a lifter would be wise to agree that conditioning work deserves a place in a year's training program, and the further along in a lifter's training journey, the more it probably matters to include.

Having said this, conditioning is usually viewed as training that can primarily improve and strengthen three key components of the 11 elements of fitness mentioned in chapter 1: cardiorespiratory capacity, muscular endurance, and body composition.

Training designed to get and keep the heart rate up for an extended time will pay dividends in the form of improving a trainee's work capacity, reducing the amount of time needed to recover (a by-product of improved muscular endurance and increased cardiorespiratory capacity), and facilitating fat loss. In the name of health, these should be reasons alone to perform conditioning work. There are several ways to approach conditioning, with or without the use of external loading.

Low-intensity steady-state (LISS) cardio is probably the most typical and most old-school method for conditioning training. It relies on the aerobic energy system and keeps the heart rate in the bottom end of the spectrum, intensity wise. Most commonly, trainees perform cardio at around 60 to

65 percent of their max heart rate. To find that percentage, the calculation is simple: 226 − age × 0.65. This means that for a 34-year-old athlete, 65 percent of their max heart rate would be 125 beats per minute. Across certification programs and exercise physiology textbooks throughout the fitness industry, this has been the guide for aerobic training and heart rate work that will trigger the utilization of carbohydrate and fat for a gradual energy burn.

Interval training takes advantage of the ATP energy source and the body's anaerobic system. This type of training is equivalent to doing something explosive, fast, and intense for a brief duration and countering it with something much lower in intensity and pace for a period to follow. A trainee would alternate these methods for a given time. An example is a three-quarter speed sprint for 10 seconds, followed by a walk for 30 seconds. Substantial research supports the idea that this kind of training can improve a trainee's rate of metabolism, which can have a lasting effect on fat loss.

Metabolic finishers often use weights, or at the very least, body weight, as a form of resistance while the athlete performs one movement (or a collection of movements) in succession, with little to no rest. This type of training is done at the end of a weight training workout, usually in an attempt to replace postworkout cardio in its more conventional forms. Common examples of metabolic finishers include sled sprint pushes or drags over a distance of 25 to 50 yards or meters, alternating between work and fairly short rest intervals (around 60-90 seconds). A lifter would usually perform this for a set window of time, such as 10 to 15 minutes. Another example is the classic inverse ladder of push-ups and chin-ups. To perform this, a lifter starts with 1 push-up, superset with 10 chin-ups. Without resting, the lifter then performs 2 push-ups and only 9 chin-ups. Then 3 push-ups and 8 chin-ups. This relative progression continues until the lifter performs 10 push-ups and 1 chin-up. This can be repeated two or three times, with 90 seconds to 2 minutes of rest between total rounds.

Classic circuit training is different from the conventional training methods discussed in this book thus far. Most of the talk to this point has been about strength movements and potentially the use of supersets, whereas circuit training involves three or more exercises performed back to back, with no rest. Of course, in these cases, the amount of weight by percentage points needs to be reduced compared with what an athlete would lift in a straight set involving no other exercises, for the same number of reps.

Sprinting is the purest form of anaerobic training in the universe—and a subcategory of metabolic training when placed under the fitness umbrella. It involves the greatest amount of muscles working together at the peak of their output, and for this reason, despite its effectiveness in creating a better conditioned human body, it requires a deep dive into technique. Many overlook the fact that just like any loaded exercise, there are form require-ments to be learned and perfected in order to avoid injury.

In keeping with the theme of this book, what matters most is that any conditioning training be regarded with the baseline of body type specificity held in first regard. For those reasons, it's worth considering a couple of truths to begin.

Truth: Real Life Requires More Muscular Endurance Than Pure Strength

This may be the only place you read a statement like this.

Using real life as our guide, the hard truth of the matter is this: We need strength a whole lot in our daily lives to make things easier, but most life demands that require strength also require muscular endurance. That's a truth that gets swept under the rug in the strength and conditioning world, in favor of heavy efforts, three-rep PRs, and a one-dimensional view of progression.

Think about this logically: We don't help someone move furniture or even carry all our groceries by picking them up for three seconds and putting them back down. In both examples, we're under tension for extended periods, and we'd be remiss to overlook that and not train for higher reps in the weight room to benefit our endurance. We don't need to say this, but it's good for our heart too. It may be a sign to zero in on this aspect of fitness in order to get into better shape.

Many coaches will say that lifting weights for higher reps makes a lifter more prone to injury because of increasing fatigue within a set. In the case of training methodologies that have you racing the clock, that's true. That's a primary reason why injuries are prevalent in many of the high-intensity fit-ness and conditioning programs that have become popular in recent years. But sets of 10 to 12 or even 15 reps of a compound movement (like a squat, deadlift, overhead press, or bench press) shouldn't be outside the vocabulary of a recreational lifter who has health and wellness first in mind, *along* with building muscle and adding strength.

The factor no one seems to mention is that the implement needs to be significantly lighter to make this happen. That in itself can spare the joints and connective tissue from plenty of stress, which is something longtime, experienced lifters eventually need to start thinking about. Moreover, assum-ing adequate rest and good form are in check, it's rare to see a lifter injure themselves during a set of 10 reps at 70 percent of their max, compared with a set of 2 or 3 reps at 90 percent.

Truth: Many Conditioning Training Protocols Do Not Take into Account the Size of the Individual

Admittedly, this truth will dominate the majority of this chapter. It's more work for a larger body to move a weight from point A to point B.

Nine times out of 10, generic "difficult" conditioning workout directives—especially for metabolic finishers—will ask a lifter to move a certain percentage of their max for some defined rep range, performed within a time constraint or with a certain amount of prescribed rest. Since you know from reading this book that *work performed* matters much more than *load lifted*—especially where conditioning and fitness are concerned—it's worth rethinking the narrative.

Remember what we said in chapter 2: Smaller lifters typically possess more relative strength, whereas larger lifters typically possess more absolute strength. It's an important distinction. It means lifters should be choosing conditioning workouts wisely. A workout involving 60 percent of a trainee's max squat for reps and short rest periods may equate to 185 pounds (85 kg) for a well-trained lifter who weighs 160 pounds (73 kg), but that could be 275 pounds (125 kg) for a lifter who weighs 240 pounds (109 kg). The bigger lifter not only has to handle a heavier implement but also has to move that implement a greater distance, assuming they are also taller. That means more work, according to its literal definition (work = force × distance). Asking a lifter to do this with the same short rest intervals as a small lifter is unrealistic and will leave the bigger lifters unable to complete the prescribed workout very early on.

This is a reality that plagues many taller and heavier lifters, and it can also falsely suggest that the lifter's conditioning and fitness levels are lower than they actually are. The truth of the matter is that it simply takes more energy to run a larger body, and that must be respected.

With energy expenditure in mind, this is what we advise big and tall lifters: Chances are, mixing big-lift percentage work (of 1RM) with high reps and fixed low rest intervals is a recipe for injury, not because of a lack of strength or capability but because of under-recovery. There's nothing wrong with doing higher-rep work, as you'll see shortly—but it's important to make the right choice. Give your body the rest and recovery it needs between sets instead of holding to 45-second guidelines.

For those who still want to time their rest intervals, at the very least be more generous with the rest assigned between sets of those big movements. Leaving the low rest periods to accessory movements performed on machines or with dumbbells can allow a larger lifter to keep the focus on technique where it matters most: under the biggest loads, during the biggest lifts.

Considerations for Low-Intensity Steady-State Cardio

Since this method is more straightforward and offers up machine-based training tools like the treadmill or elliptical, it's a simple matter of calculation (described earlier) to find a trainee's 60 or 65 percent max heart rate. A trainee will then adjust the speed, resistance, or incline of the apparatus accordingly to maintain the intensity goal for a set period. Spending 30 to 40 minutes with the heart rate elevated to this level can yield excellent benefits for the cardiovascular system and heart health. For a smaller, lighter lifter, chances are the speed, resistance, or incline needed will end up being slightly higher than what's needed for a larger, heavier lifter to attain the same result.

In the case of the rowing machine, a lifter can focus primarily on movement efficiency. However, it's important to note one guideline: A lifter should not use the metric of time per 500 meters, or strokes per minute, in order to gauge performance. This is where taller, longer-limbed lifters have a slight advantage in the world of training. In the actual sport of rowing, you'll find many rowers possessing tall, long-limbed bodies because it optimizes the distance covered per stroke and affects the speed of the boat (along with the efficiency in reaching and maintaining that speed). Taking fewer strokes to cover the same distance means a slower frequency at each joint and the savings of some crucial energy. All of this to say, it's going to be easier to have a faster time per 500 meters as a 6-foot-5 athlete than as a 5-foot-4 athlete (figure 13.1a-b). A training expectation or directive of maintaining 2:10 per 500 meters (as an example) in a 3-kilometer row will be much more realistic for a trained taller lifter than it would be for a trained shorter lifter. Like any piece of equipment, the rowing machine needs to be used with proper technique, and it's not exempt simply because it's a piece of cardio equipment. Optimal rowing requires a chain of coordinated actions, and receiving initial coaching would be

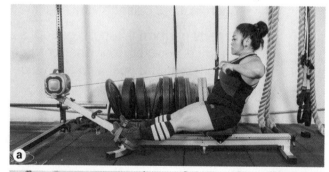

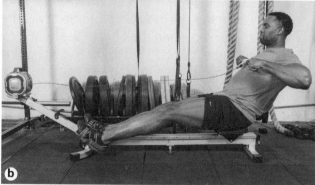

FIGURE 13.1   Rowing machine for a shorter lifter *(a)*, and a taller person *(b)*.

very beneficial to a lifter learning to use it, in order to prevent injury or over-reliance on the wrong muscle groups to perform the action.

Aside from machine-based cardio methods, lifters can mimic the demands of steady-state cardio training by using light implements and, once again, putting aside the idea of lifting percentages and instead thinking about using a light load that enables them to remain in motion for the entire duration.

Alternating Turkish Get-Ups

On its own, getting down on the ground and up off the ground is more physi-cally demanding and aerobically challenging than many give it credit for. Using a light kettlebell or dumbbell as loading can be the perfect challenge for a lifter without being too overbearing. The Turkish get-up is a unique choice compared with other up-and-down exercises, such as burpees, because they are typically performed at a slower, more controlled pace to keep one eye on safety while also incorporating the mobility, stability, and general athletic improvement of various structures of the body:

- Strength endurance and stability of the shoulder capsule
- Shoulder, hip, and thoracic spine mobility
- Abdominal and oblique strength
- Posterior chain activation
- Coordination, balance, and spatial awareness

To properly perform a Turkish get-up, a lifter starts by lying on their back with one knee bent, so that one foot is flat on the ground and the other leg is straight out. The goal is to get "wide" by spreading out the arms and straight leg.

Holding a kettlebell (with the weight on the outside of the forearm) or dumbbell in the same-side hand as the bent leg, the next step is to extend the arm so it's pointing straight up to the roof (figure 13.2a). A lifter should keep the eyes focused on the bell and knuckles facing the ceiling. These rules should never be compromised.

Using the abs in kind of a sit-up style, the lifter presses into the floor with the free elbow and the heel of the bent leg in order to get into a seated posi-tion (figure 13.2b). It's okay to use a bit of momentum to make this possible.

Making sure the loaded arm remains straight, the next step once position-ing has been established while resting on the elbow is to press once more with the grounded arm until the lifter is resting only on the hand and sitting upright (figure 13.2c).

Once in the seated position, the lifter digs in with the planted hand and heel to create a high bridge (figure 13.2d). Squeezing the glutes and brac-ing the core are essential to raise the hips high enough off the ground for proper clearance for the next phase—getting the free (straight) leg to travel under (figure 13.2e).

The lifter then carefully brings that leg through the underpass by bending the knee and pulling it through. That knee is planted on the ground, under the body, freeing up the ability to release the grounded hand and get tall in a half-kneeling position (figure 13.2f).

Finally, the only step left is to stand tall, with the weight directly overhead. Still keeping the eyes up, the lifter focuses on carefully standing without letting the elbow bend (figure 13.2g). This may be a more difficult than it

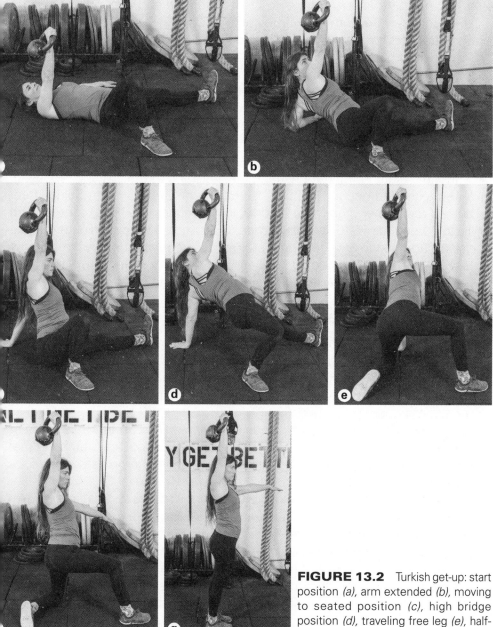

FIGURE 13.2 Turkish get-up: start position (a), arm extended (b), moving to seated position (c), high bridge position (d), traveling free leg (e), half-kneeling position (f), finish (g).

sounds, which is why the weight chosen at the beginning to groove this skill matters most.

Remember—the get-up also involves getting back down. Since the ground won't go anywhere, keeping the eyes up and learning to reverse the previous actions by feel and not by looking down is an invaluable skill to master. A break in focus can cause the bell to fall. First, the lifter puts the same knee (the one opposite the working arm) gently down to the ground, under control. The free hand is planted to the side of the body, not behind it. This gives the body enough space to create a bridge and pick up the planted knee so it can travel through to its original straight-leg position, the way it started. The lifter slowly kicks it through and then plants the hips down to the ground under control.

Next, the planted arm slides outward until the elbow contacts the ground, and then the shoulders and back are allowed to follow to the ground too. By this point the lifter should be lying in the starting position.

That's a lot of steps, but it looks more daunting in writing than in practice. It takes only a few reps to get very good at this exercise, and a recommended protocol is simply alternating between hands (i.e., getting up and back down with the weight in the right hand, then switching to the left and repeating) for an extended period. The time is contingent on the weight being lifted, but we recommend no more than 25 to 35 pounds (12-15 kg) for men and 10 to 20 pounds (5-10 kg) for women. Starting with two 5-minute rounds, using a 90-second break of complete rest between rounds, is a good litmus test for a lifter's conditioning level and allows them to focus on an evenly paced effort without having a set amount of reps to perform.

Every Minute on the Minute Training

Training every minute on the minute (EMOM) is a very demanding method that builds conditioning. The athlete simply starts the clock and performs a set number of reps while the clock runs. Once finished with the set, the remainder of that minute can be dedicated to rest. The next set begins at the top of the next minute.

A typical EMOM set usually ends up giving a lifter 35 to 45 seconds of rest before the next set begins. The good thing about this method is that a lifter can do the EMOM style for as long or as little time as preferred, as their conditioning allows.

EMOM training for the sake of conditioning works best with larger movements, since the body's total expenditure will lead to a greater increase in heart rate and need for recovery time compared with a smaller lift. Exercises like the pull-up, squat, deadlift, overhead press, and bench press are all fair game for applying this method—but special measures must be taken.

First, remember that these are big lifts for the intention of prolonged effort. With that said, choosing a suitable weight should not be based off rep range percentages. We've found that regardless of size, trained individuals do well to base things off of percentages of their body weight instead, because the selected weight represents something much more realistic for multiple sets. See table 13.1 for sample EMOM suggestions.

TABLE 13.1   Sample EMOM Suggestions

Exercise	Percentage of body weight
Bench press	60%
Squat	80%
Deadlift	100% (body-weight equivalent)
Overhead press	40%
Chin-up	100% (body-weight equivalent, if applicable)

Athlete size, leverages, and time under tension per rep is where things differ, and that comes in the form of repetitions performed. As an example, in a 20-minute EMOM squat effort, a lifter who's bigger and taller may choose three reps whereas a shorter, lighter lifter may choose five. Likewise, a shorter-armed lifter may opt for five or six reps in a bench press EMOM compared with a long-armed lifter's three or four. Considering the amount of time it takes for the phosphocreatine system—the immediate energy source muscles rely on to access short-term bursts of power and strength—to be depleted (between 10 and 15 seconds), we recommend that the amount of work performed not exceed the time window, allowing ample time for partial rejuvenation of the muscles' ATP for the next set.

The idea of training every minute on the minute may look easy, especially when considering the submaximal loading being recommended, but if an honest starting weight is chosen and the clock is being obeyed, all lifters should feel quite aerobically and muscularly fatigued around set number eight. For big-lift EMOMs, we recommend a 15-to 20-minute duration. If the lifter completes all the reps in 20 minutes, increasing the weight or reps performed per set by a comfortable increment is recommended. Once again, the good thing about this technique is that it backs off on the amount of weight being lifted and the number of reps performed (relative to the most a lifter can do under normal circumstances) and counters that with very short rest intervals.

A lifter can do two exercises using the EMOM method in the same workout to make for a full-fledged conditioning session, but they would do well to make sure their choices are not competing movements. In other words, pairing the strict press with the bench press or the squat with the deadlift (as examples) wouldn't be wise, since many of the same muscles would be involved, which increases risk for the second exercise and may reduce or compromise performance.

Considerations for High-Intensity Interval Training

Since high-intensity interval training (HIIT) methods involve intermittent bouts of hard work (typically with much less rest time), it's a safer, smarter approach to work with little to no weight if possible. In truth, countless methods of HIIT can be used as examples, but we'd like to compare and contrast smaller, lighter lifters with bigger, heavier individuals once again, using the Tabata method. Tabata training is one of the most popular forms of HIIT conditioning in the fitness world, but sadly, it's often misapplied from its true purpose and execution.

Tabata-style workouts are designed to bring athletes toward their anaerobic threshold. They consist of 20 seconds of work followed by 10 seconds of rest, repeated for eight rounds per exercise. When done correctly, each exercise lasts a total of 3:50, and then the athlete moves on to the next exercise. This is the purist version for effective muscle breakdown, but some people like using a circuit-style method that cycles among various exercises for each 20-second burst. Tabata training targets the anaerobic energy system. The 20 seconds of work should be more than enough to bring a working muscle to complete fatigue, with very little time allowance to rejuvenate ATP between rounds.

That means each effort should be made with purpose to exploit the depletion of ATP and push to the limits of the anaerobic threshold. Every effort should be explosive. It's better to pause during the running time and regather for a few seconds if that means the next effort will be explosive rather than slow and weak. If a person is still moving perfectly fine by the fifth or sixth set out of eight, they haven't gone hard enough to properly execute the set. This method should really break the working muscles down and produce a significant amount of lactic burn.

A second by-product of Tabata training is the phenomenon of EPOC: excess postworkout oxygen consumption. The anaerobic effort of the Tabata method places the working muscles in an oxygen debt, which the body needs time to make up. It's the reason sprinters who perform a max-effort 100-meter dash for just 10 seconds breathe heavily for minutes to follow. This state encourages an increased metabolic demand, which can lead to fat loss while training the fast-twitch muscle fibers of the body. The following exercise options for the Tabata method work well:

- Squats (body weight or very lightly loaded goblet squats)
- Lunges (body weight)
- Push-ups
- Inverted rows
- Bent-over rows (very lightly loaded)

- Sit-ups
- Mountain climbers
- Assault bike or Airdyne bike
- Dumbbell neutral-grip overhead press (very lightly loaded)
- Deep squat jumps (body weight)
- Medicine ball slams

With all of this said, the Tabata method should definitely be reserved for intermediate or advanced lifters who have a good base of general conditioning. It's far less purposeful to perform these at half the effort, and it breaches their intended use. But the smaller, lighter lifter will be at a marked advantage when performing the Tabata method for two reasons: (1) Smaller levers equal a faster frequency, and (2) a shorter range of motion equals less work, meaning a faster rate of recovery per effort. Larger individuals need to pay attention to recovery time to get the same benefits without an early burnout.

Big Lifters and Tabata Training

Simply reversing the work-to-rest ratio can be a saving grace for big lifters in search of the benefits that Tabata training has to offer. Working as hard as possible for 10 seconds and then resting for 20 seconds, with the same eight-set duration per exercise, can be the difference maker that allows a heavier or taller lifter to make it through an entire workout, with all things equal.

A lifter shouldn't be using weights to scale for their body weight during a Tabata workout. For any exercises in the list of Tabata options that involve external loading, 10 pounds (5 kg) per hand is more than enough for a full-grown adult who's well conditioned.

Furthermore, following one exercise with another one that works synergistic muscles could compromise form and technique. Performing a Tabata-method squat followed by a Tabata-method lunge, or a Tabata-method sit-up followed by Tabata-method mountain climbers, would be detrimental to the second exercise. Allowing some time for a muscle group in question to recover by making the next exercise focus on a very different prime mover is recommended, such as pairing a Tabata-method overhead press with a Tabata-method stationary lunge.

Sprinting (and Sprinting as HIIT)

Sprinting is very commonly employed as a conditioning method, and especially when placed in an interval setting (also known as tempo sprint work), it can be very athletically demanding. Many make the mistake of thinking that, since sprinting is free of external load and based on an individual's abilities and nothing more, it's a fairly foolproof exercise for safe, intense training. But like any exercise in the gym, the act of sprinting requires plenty of attention to detail to ensure safety.

The bigger and heavier the athlete, the more force the athlete can potentially apply against a resistance. Vigorous exercises like sprinting require extremely aggressive contractions both concentrically and eccentrically, especially if a lifter is not in a regular habit of getting out on the track to train. And for the record, once weekly during the summer doesn't cut it. The difference between a track athlete and a lifter who likes to sprint for conditioning is that the athlete spends 15 hours per week on the track and 3 in the weight room. Lifters might spend 10 or so hours per week in the weight room but only 1 hour per week on the track. That difference, especially when coupled with being older in adulthood, is a major reason to keep safety top of mind when on the track as a recreational sprinter. If they are not careful, sprinting could open lifters up to straining or even tearing muscles, regardless of technique. Here are a few recommendations to ensure that doesn't happen.

• *First, always leave something in the tank.* It's important to acknowledge the difference between sprinting for competition and sprinting for conditioning and its athletic and health benefits. A trained sprinter knows there's a huge difference between sprinting at 90 percent of max speed versus going full tilt. To the onlooker, there wouldn't be much difference in speed (or even in a clocked sprint time), but sticking with 90 percent output will significantly encourage more relaxation and fluidity.

• *Stick with longer sprint distances.* Distances of 30 and 40 yards or meters encourage a lifter to tighten up and get to the line in a mad dash. Sprinting at 85 or 90 percent of maximum speed is still sprinting. Allowing more rest time between sets of 100- or 150-meter sprints (versus shorter rest and 40-meter repeats) will not only help a lifter open up their stride but also provide more time under tension and really zero in on conditioning.

For a good sprint workout, performing proper mobility drills, stretches, and warm-up sprint drills like A skips, running A's, butt kicks, and carioca are important to start things off. Here is an example of a longer sprint workout that is in keeping with what's recommended: After some warm-up drills and a few preparatory sprints of 30 or 40 yards or meters (resting as long as needed), the lifter performs 2 × 80 meters, 2 × 100 meters, and finally 4 × 120 meters. The lifter walks back to the starting line between reps; an additional 30- to 60-second rest on top of this is acceptable before repeating.

• *Avoid using the treadmill.* For the most part, sprinting on a machine that has a belt speed limit of just 12 miles per hour (19 km/h) isn't sprinting. Elite athletes reach top-end speeds of nearly 30 miles per hour (48 km/h) during the 100-meter dash. Even though a lifter may not be elite, it's still reasonable to think many can move faster than 12 miles per hour over ground.

Also, the moving belt on a treadmill is pulling the athlete's leg through the motion instead of the athlete relying on an active hip extension. It's best to learn good form by sprinting outside.

• *Use a falling start rather than exploding from a dead stop.* Taking off from a completely static position like a three-point stance or from starting blocks requires deep hip and knee flexion and is a very aggressive ask for your body; that's an easy way to strain a muscle that's not quite conditioned enough to be in track shape in the first few strides. Using a falling start instead—where a runner starts tall and slowly lowers into a staggered-stance half squat, while letting natural momentum and gravity pull them forward until they have no choice but to take off—is a safety method we endorse for a gradual change in joint angle that tends to feel much more natural and less jarring. To be extra safe, a lifter should start sprinting from a 5- to 10-stride jog.

• *When sprinting for tempo work or HIIT, the same principles apply as when performing gym-based exercises for the same purposes.* Simply put, the ability to work at a certain level of effort will need to be compromised, and there is no disputing this. That's the reason why back-to-back 100-meter sprints with only 30 seconds of rest in between will not result in the same time performance. Knowing this, a lifter who uses a typical HIIT or tempo sprinting protocol (like sprinting the straightaways of the track and walking, skipping, or jogging the corners) will be wise to use a much reduced pace during the sprints themselves; around 75 percent of max effort is smarter than 90 or 95 percent.

Hill Sprints

Doing sprints up a reasonable incline can fix faulty sprinting mechanics since an athlete will be working against physics in a more direct way. Getting up to the top of the hill without wasted energy forces a lifter to use more linear force production, a greater arm drive, and a higher knee lift in order to get from point A to point B. Moreover, other compensations like rotating excessively through the trunk or using short, choppy strides will show up very early on. In addition, since uphill sprinting is more of a climb than a run, it has less impact on the joints. Sprinting is likely not as high on the priority list as lifting weights, so including hill work versus flat ground work can be a very important factor to keep strength training exercises like squats, lunges, and deadlifts from being compromised by residual joint pain.

Using the hill sprint as a HIIT method could look something like this: 16 × 40 yards or meters at 80 to 85 percent of top speed. A slow walk down the hill, plus an additional 30 seconds of rest between sprint starts, is recommended.

Sprinting and hill sprinting can be used as their own workout or as a HIIT or metabolic finisher after a strength training workout in the gym. Just know that because of the neurological demand (sprinting is purely fast-twitch dominant, meaning the high-threshold motor units will be hit the hardest), it's worthwhile to temper performance expectations since many of those muscles will have been fatigued lifting heavy weights and using the same energy systems.

Sled and Prowler Pushing and Pulling

The prowler or sled has been mentioned as an option for metabolic conditioning, but it has even greater utility as a tool for sprint training. Similar to hill sprints, pushing or towing an object from one place to another using the body typically lends to a self-adjustment of form and technique in the name of locomotive efficiency. The good news about using sleds for conditioning is that they facilitate loaded work with unloaded eccentric phases. The muscles of the lower body have to move the heavy load only on each push of the stride; for the leg to recover to its original position, no resistance exists (figure 13.3). As you learned in earlier chapters, eccentric-free training can create a window for higher work volume since they can cause less muscle trauma.

Using the sled or prowler for conditioning allows for versatility; this piece of equipment can be used at a slow pace with lighter weight loaded for steady-state training, or it can be used at a faster pace with heavier weight (and shorter distances and overall duration) as a HIIT method.

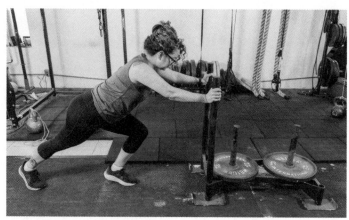

FIGURE 13.3   Sled or prowler stand.

Considerations for Circuit Training

Choosing appropriate circuits for circuit training requires a lifter to think about a number of factors, including some already discussed:

- Movements that are friendly to the body and joints depending on body type
- Movements that don't involve competing muscle groups
- Movements that aren't hindered by nonfocal factors such as grip strength, balance, or low back fatigue

The third point is very interesting. When a lifter's ability to have a good workout is held prisoner to a part of the lift that shouldn't be of concern in the name of performance, problems could arise and prove very frustrating. One example would be a circuit that looks like the following:

1. Barbell deadlift: 10 reps
2. Body-weight pull-up: 10 reps
3. Hang clean: 5 reps
4. Dumbbell walking lunge: 20 strides
5. Hammer curl: 10 reps

Although this seems like it would be a great workout and a definite way to get conditioned in a hurry, the commonality among all these movements is that they're grip intensive. Each of them relies on a strong hold on the implement in question, and a lifter can count on their grip to fatigue and fail them faster than any muscle group, especially by the second or third round of work. A better idea would be to choose a combination of pull-based and push-based exercises for the upper body that may even involve an open and closed hand position.

Taller or longer-legged lifters would be smart to consider which compound movements based on their biomechanics tend to cause more than normal amounts of stress to key regions like the shoulders, knees, or lumbar spine. Choosing exercises in a set-and-rest fashion may be something a lifter would normally be able to get away with, free of any unwanted pain or discomfort, but arranging things into a circuit with reduced rest may compound what was once a minor issue. Take this example in the case of a lifter with long legs and a short torso:

1. Conventional barbell deadlift
2. Overhead press
3. Bent-over row
4. Body-weight dip
5. Goblet squat

In this case, the lifter would benefit from choosing at least two smaller movements that are more isolated in nature, considering all five of these movements, because the geometrical angles assumed or the range of motion to create a full rep, will place a whole lot of loading on either the lumbar spine or shoulder capsule. As great as each of these movements is, they may not be as great for a lifter of this body type when arranged back to back with no rest.

Choose Weight Wisely

By this point in the chapter, it's no secret that conditioning training and rep range percentages don't go hand in hand. Dedicating one or more lifts in a circuit to body-weight effort or very light loads can do plenty to keep the heart rate elevated while sparing the joints and connective tissue of additional loading that can break down technique in the presence of fatigue. For example, if back squats are originally part of a circuit that involves two other big lifts, swapping to a goblet squat may be a major difference maker. In the case of a goblet squat, a lifter will be limited by the weight of a dumbbell, which can very well be lighter than the amount of weight they would squat with a bar.

Moreover, choosing exercises that allow the aerobic system to be trained while still moving a reasonably loaded implement brings credence to the idea of revisiting the definition of power from chapter 1: the intersection of strength and speed. In the case of power training, the lifter will be using an implement that can be properly accelerated, rather than a weight that will move slowly because the load is too heavy. This can be mimicked from a conditioning standpoint by choosing exercises that use lighter loads but still serve the purpose of training explosiveness and developing speed and power. Such movements can also be performed for higher reps, within a window of 15 or so seconds:

- Kettlebell swing
- Medicine ball slam
- Medicine ball wall throw (forward or sideways)
- Kettlebell or dumbbell snatch
- Squat jump
- Weight vest push-up or plyometric push-ups
- Jump or switch split squat

The good news is that all these exercises allow muscular endurance to be trained effectively since they enable the use of high rep ranges. Sets of 10 to 20 reps using lower weight where applicable is recommended.

Complexes for Conditioning in a Poorly Equipped Space

If a lifter is training in a small space or has few equipment options, the complex is a smart conditioning tool to put to use, mainly because it requires only a single piece of equipment—be it a pair of kettlebells, a barbell, or a pair of dumbbells (as examples). To perform a complex, a lifter does a series of exercises in succession without putting the weight down between. The complex takes on the identity of one massive set, which in turn increases time under tension, valuable not only for conditioning but also for grip strength, because the lifter will be holding on to the implement for a prolonged period. In the case of smaller, lighter lifters specifically, complexes can provide a challenge that brief rests between exercises in a circuit or other conditioning workout may not.

With complexes, it's important to play toward an athlete's weaknesses rather than their strengths. A complex of a deadlift, bent-over row, clean, and overhead press, for example, will be limited in weight by the strength of the overhead press, because that's typically the weakest of these movements. With that said, modifying the complex by simply reducing the number of reps required for the weakest lift is the smart way to go rather than reducing weight overall and making the other three movements suffer in terms of loading.

Beyond that, since a lifter is meant to go from one movement right into the next with no breaks, it makes things easier if there's some form of progression through the chain so that the exercises somewhat flow together. For example, it would be a real hassle going from a deadlift straight into a back squat using a barbell, since the lifter would have to first deadlift the bar, then clean it up to shoulder level, then press it over to load it on the back. Compare that complex with one comprising the deadlift, row, clean, push press, and back squat, which makes for much smoother transitions from exercise to exercise.

As you can see, conditioning can take on many forms. And in 7,000 words, we're only scratching the surface of the options available, even despite discrepancies in leverages or size. When training an individual, it's important to choose the right conditioning tools for the lifter so they last the test of time in the gym and can be adequately challenged without burning out.

Chapter 14

Sample Workouts

The nuances of a workout are completely dependent on the goals of the athlete. A physique program will look different from a powerlifting program, which will look different from an endurance program, which will look different from a sport-specific program, and so forth. Furthermore, programming for a beginning lifter will be different from that of an experienced lifter. Sets, reps, exercise selection, and volume all depend on the goals and abilities of the athlete.

That said, we are providing some sample generalized workouts as examples of how an athlete might bring together different training components in order to best meet their needs. This is by no means a mandate or set in stone: These are simply a reference point from which to start.

UPPER BODY TRAINING, BENCH PRESS FOCUS: LONG ARMS

Exercise	Page number	Thumbnail
Pin press	110	
Bench press (slow, eccentric tempo)	108	
Single-arm dumbbell row	156	
Cable crossover	198	
Narrow-stance push-up	194	
Pallof press	176	

UPPER BODY TRAINING, OVERHEAD FOCUS: SHORT ARMS

Exercise	Page number	Thumbnail
Overhead press	126	
Push-ups on hex dumbbells or push-up handles	193	
Sternum pull-up	146	
Flexed arm hang	137	
Band-assisted wheel rollout	173	

TOTAL BODY CONDITIONING: BIG ALL OVER

Exercise	Page number	Thumbnail
Box squat	100	
Medium sumo barbell deadlift	77	
Ring inverted row	160	
Dumbbell bench press	119	
Band-assisted pull-up	144	
Weighted carries	179	

LOWER BODY TRAINING, SQUAT FOCUS: LONG FEMURS

Exercise	Page number	Thumbnail
Back squat (pause for 2 seconds at the bottom of the movement)	36	
Heels-elevated dumbbell or kettlebell squat	91	
Walking lunge	211	
Copenhagen plank	225	
Nordic curl hip hinge	217	

LOWER BODY TRAINING, DEADLIFT FOCUS: LONG LEGS, SHORT ARMS

Exercise	Page number	Thumbnail
Trap bar deadlift, high handle	71	
Eccentric Nordic curl	216	
Rear-foot-elevated split squat	222	
Cable pull-through	230	
Reverse hyperextensions	221	

UPPER BODY TRAINING, BENCH PRESS FOCUS: LONG ARMS

Exercise	Page number	Thumbnail
Bench press	108	
Pin press	110	
Dumbbell snatch	206	
Plyometric push-up	192	

UPPER BODY TRAINING, PULL FOCUS: LONG ARMS

Exercise	Page number	Thumbnail
Barbell deadlift	32	
Pendlay row	164	
Eccentric chin-up	139	
Wide-grip seated row	163	
Inchworms	173	

UPPER BODY TRAINING, PULL FOCUS: SMALL HANDS

Exercise	Page number	Thumbnail
Barbell deadlift (straps) OR Eccentric-free deadlift	32	
Neutral-grip chin-up	142	
Ring inverted row	160	
Band-resisted row	167	
Lat pull-down	208	
Hanging knee raise (straps)	178	

Everything you've read in this chapter drives home the point made in the introductory chapters: The big lifts are important to learn and master—even with allowance for variability depending on body type and anthropometry. But mastering and practicing the big lifts shouldn't be at the expense of important assistance exercises that will round out a lifter's training program and add much-needed depth to exercise prescription. In turn, these added exercises will improve the body's overall capability and athleticism, which serves the greater purpose of covering more components of fitness (to transcend the skills built in only five or six major movements). Understanding the needs of the individual body type truly sets the framework and cornerstone as a starting point for safe and effective strength training.

Implementing all the information about big lifts into a program that includes several exercises, prescribed reps, sets, and rest is the true practical application of the science behind body type specificity. It's a foolproof approach to building a strong body that functions like a well-oiled machine—one that won't break down after short-term use!

References

Chapter 1

Aouadi, R., M.C. Jlid MC, R. Khalifa et al. 2012. Association of anthropometric qualities with vertical jump performance in elite male volleyball players. *Journal of Sports Medicine and Physical Fitness* 52 (1): 11-17.

Azcorra, H., M.I. Varela-Silva, L. Rodriguez, B. Bogin, and F. Dickinson. 2013. Nutritional status of Maya children, their mothers, and their grandmothers residing in the City of Merica, Mexico: Revisiting the leg-length hypothesis. *American Journal of Human Biology* 25:659-665. https://doi.org/10.1002/ajhb.22427.

Bishop, C., A. Turner, and P. Read. 2018. Effects of inter-limb asymmetries on physical and sports performance: A systematic review. *Journal of Sports Sciences* 36 (10): 1135-1144. https://doi.org/10.1080/02640414.2017.1361894.

Bogin, B., & M.I. Varela-Silva. 2010. Leg length, body proportion, and health: A review with a note on beauty. *International Journal of Environmental Research and Public Health* 7:1047-1075. http://dx.doi.org/10.3390/ijerph7031047.

Epstein, D. 2013. *The Sports Gene*, 117-120. New York: Penguin Books.

Fryar, C., et al. 2018. National Health Statistics reports: Mean body height, weight, waist circumference and body mass index among adults: United States, 1999-2000 through 2015-16. December 20, 2018. www.cdc.gov/nchs/data/nhsr/nhsr122-508.pdf.

Keogh, J.W.L., P.A. Hume, S.N. Pearson, and P. Mellow. 2007. Anthropometric dimensions of male powerlifters of varying body mass, *Journal of Sports Sciences* 25 (12): 1365-1376. https://doi.org/10.1080/02640410601059630.

Keogh, J.W.L., P.A. Hume, S.N. Pearson, and P.J. Mellow. 2009. Can absolute and proportional anthropometric characteristics distinguish stronger and weaker powerlifters? *Journal of Strength and Conditioning Research* 23 (8): 2256-2265. https://doi.org/10.1519/JSC.0b013e3181b8d67a.

Kuznetsova, Z.M., S.A. Kuznetsov, Y.D. Ovchinnikov, and P.V. Golovko. 2018. Analysis of the morphological-functional indices connection degree in throwing among athletes. Педагогико-психологические и медико-биологические проблемы физической культуры и спорта 13 (2): 44-50. https://cyberleninka.ru/article/n/analysis-of-the-morphological-functional-indices-connection-degree-in-throwing-among-athletes.

Musser, L.J., J. Garhammer, R. Rozenek, J.A. Crussemeyer, and E.M. Vargas. 2014. Anthropometry and barbell trajectory in the snatch lift for elite women weightlifters. *Journal of Strength and Conditioning Research* 28 (6): 1636-1648. https://doi.org/10.1519/JSC.0000000000000450.

Nevill, A.M., S. Oxford, and M.J. Duncan. 2015. Optimal body size and limb-length ratios associated with 100-m PB swim speeds. *Medicine and Science in Sports and Exercise* 47 (8): 1714-1718.

Purnell, J.Q. 2018. Definitions, classification, and epidemiology of obesity. In *Endotext*, edited by K.R. Feingold, B. Anawalt, A. Boyce, et al. www.ncbi.nlm.nih.gov/books/NBK279167.

Roser, M., C. Appel, C., and H. Ritchie. 2013. Human height. Our World in Data. https://ourworldindata.org/human-height.

Ruff, C. 2002. Variation in human body size and shape. *Annual Review of Anthropology* 31:211-232. https://doi.org/10.1146/annurev.anthro.31.040402.085407.

Sarvestan, J., V. Riedel, Z. Gonosová, P. Linduška, and M. Přidalová. 2019. Relationship between anthropometric and strength variables and maximal throwing velocity in female junior handball players: A pilot study. *Acta Gymnica* 49 (3): 132-137. https://doi.org/10.5507/ag.2019.012.

Top End Sports. 2015. Anthropometric measurements of 100m Olympic champions. Updated December 2015. www.topendsports.com/events/summer/science/athletics-100m.htm.

Vidal Pérez, D., J.M. Martínez-Sanz, A. Ferriz-Valero, V. 2021. Gómez-Vicente, and E. Ausó. Relationship of limb lengths and body composition to lifting in weightlifting. *International Journal of Environmental Research and Public Health* 18 (2): 756. https://doi.org/10.3390/ijerph18020756.

Chapter 2

Epstein, D. 2013. *The Sports Gene*, 117-120. New York: Penguin Books.

Fryar, C., et al. 2018. National Health Statistics reports: Mean body height, weight, waist circumference and body mass index among adults: United States, 1999-2000 through 2015-16. December 20, 2018. www.cdc.gov/nchs/data/nhsr/nhsr122-508.pdf.

Roser, M., C. Appel, and H. Ritchie, H. 2013. Human height. Our World in Data. https://ourworldindata.org/human-height.

Top End Sports. 2015. Anthropometric measurements of 100m Olympic champions. Updated December 2015. www.topendsports.com/events/summer/science/athletics-100m.htm.

Chapter 3

Dickie, J.A., J.A. Faulkner, M.J. Barnes, and S.D. Lark. 2017. Electromyographic analysis of muscle activation during pull-up variations. *Journal of Electromyography and Kinesiology* 32:30-36.

DiNunzio, C., N. Porter, J. Van Scoy, D. Cordice, and R.S. McCulloch. 2018. Alterations in kinematics and muscle activation patterns with the addition of a kipping action during a pull-up activity. *Sports Biomechanics* 18 (6): 622-635. https://doi.org/10.1080/14763141.2018.1452971.

García-Ramos, A., A. Pérez-Castilla, F.J. Villar Macias, A. Latorre-Roman, J.A. Parraga, and F. Garcia-Pinillos. 2021. Differences in the one-repetition maximum and load-velocity profile between the flat and arched bench press in competitive powerlifters. *Sports Biomechanics* 20 (3): 261-273. https://doi.org/10.1080/14763141.2018.1544662.

Gardner, J.K., J.T. Chia, B.M. Peterson, and K.L. Miller. 2021. The effects of 5 weeks of leg-drive training on bench performance in recreationally-trained, college-age men. *Journal of Science in Sport and Exercise*. May 12, 2021. https://doi.org/10.1007/s42978-021-00118-0.

Lehman, G.J., D.D. Buchan, A. Lundy, N. Myers, and A. Nalborczyk. 2004. Variations in muscle activation levels during traditional latissimus dorsi weight training exercises: An experimental study. *Dynamic Medicine* 3 (4). https://doi.org/10.1186/1476-5918-3-4.

Pinto, B.L., and C.R. Dickerson. 2021. Vertical and horizontal barbell kinematics indicate differences in mechanical advantage between using an arched or flat back posture in the barbell bench press exercise. *International Journal of Sports Science & Coaching* 16 (3): 756-762. https://doi.org/10.1177/1747954120982954.

Quillen, D.M., M. Wuchner, and R. Hatch. 2004. Acute shoulder injuries. *American Family Physician* 70 (10): 1947-1954.

Williamson, T., and P. Price. 2021. A comparison of muscle activity between strict, kipping, and butterfly pull-ups. *Journal of Sport & Exercise Science* 5 (2): 149-155. https://doi.org/10.36905/jses.2021.02.08.

Wright, G.A., T.H. Delong, and G. Gehlsen. 1999. Electromyographic activity of the hamstrings during performance of the leg curl, stiff leg deadlift, and back squat movements. *Journal of Strength and Conditioning Research* 13 (2): 168-174.

Chapter 4

Bengtsson, V., L. Berglung, and U. Aasa. 2018. Narrative review of injuries in powerlifting with special reference to their association to the squat, bench press and deadlift. *BMJ Open Sport & Exercise Medicine* 4:e000382. https://doi.org/10.1136/bjmsem-2018-000382.

Chou, P.H., S.Z. Lou, S.K. Chen, H.C. Chen, T.H. Hsia, T.L. Liao, and Y.L. Chou. 2008. Elbow load during different types of bench-press exercise. *Biomedical Engineering: Applications, Basis, and Communications* 20 (3): 185-189. https://doi.org/10.4015/S1016237208000775.

Cotterman, M.L., L.A. Darby, and W.A. Skelly. 2005. Comparison of muscle force production using the Smith machine and free weights for bench press and squat exercises. *Journal of Strength and Conditioning Research* 19 (1): 169-176.

Escamilla, R.F., T.M. Lowry, D.C. Osbahr, and K.P. Speer. 2001. Biomechanical analysis of the deadlift during the 1999 Special Olympics World Games. *Medicine & Science in Sports & Exercise* 33 (8): 1345-1353. https://doi.org/10.1097/00005768-200108000-00016.

Fleisig, G.S., S.W. Barrentine, N. Zheng, R.F. Escamilla, and J.R. Andrews. 1999. Kinematic and kinetic comparison of baseball pitching among various levels of development. *Journal of Biomechanics* 32 (12): 1371-1375.

Merriam-Webster. n.d. Force. www.merriam-webster.com/dictionary/force.

Schoenfeld, B.J. 2010. Squatting kinematics and kinetics and their application to exercise performance. *Journal of Strength and Conditioning Research* 24 (12): 3497-3506.

Chapter 5

Andersen, V., M.S. Fimland, D.A. Mo, V.M. Iversen, T. Vederhus, L.R.R. Hellebø, and A.H. Saeterbakken. 2018. Electromyographic comparison of barbell deadlift, hex bar deadlift, and hip thrust exercises: A cross-over study. *Journal of Strength and Conditioning Research* 32 (3): 587-593.

Mawston, G., L. Holder, P. O'Sullivan, and M. Boocock. 2021. Flexed lumbar spine postures are associated with greater strength and efficiency than lordotic postures during a maximal lift in pain-free individuals. *Gait & Posture* 86:245-250. https://doi.org/10.1016/j.gaitpost.2021.02.029.

McGill, S., A. McDermott, and C.M. Fenwick. 2009. Comparison of different strongman events: Trunk muscle activation and lumbar spine motion, load, and stiffness. *Journal of Strength and Conditioning Research* 23 (4): 1148-1161. https://doi.org/10.1519/JSC.0b013e318198f8f7.

Swinton, P.A., A. Stewart, I. Agouris, J.W.L. Keogh, and R. Lloyd. 2011. A biomechanical analysis of straight and hexagonal barbell deadlifts using submaximal loads. *Journal of Strength and Conditioning Research* 25 (7): 2000-2009.

Chapter 6

Fuglsang, E.I., A.S. Telling, and H. Sørensen. 2017. Effect of ankle mobility and segment ratios on trunk lean in the barbell back squat. *Journal of Strength and Conditioning Research* 31 (11): 3024-3033.

Hales, M.E., B.F. Johnson, and J.T. Johnson. 2009. Kinematic analysis of the powerlifting style squat and the conventional deadlift during competition: Is there a cross-over effect between lifts? *Journal of Strength and Conditioning Research* 23 (9): 2574-2580.

Joseph, L., J. Reilly, K. Sweezey, R. Waugh, L.A. Carlson, and M.A. Lawrence. 2020. Activity of trunk and lower extremity musculature: Comparison between parallel back squats and belt squats. *Journal of Human Kinetics* 72:223-228.

McBride, J.M., J.W. Skinner, P.C. Schafer, T.L. Haines, and T.J. Kirby. 2010. Comparison of kinetic variables and muscle activity during a squat vs. a box squat. *Journal of Strength and Conditioning Research* 24 (12): 3195-3199.

Chapter 7

Bellar, D.M., L.W. Judge, T.J Patrick, and E.L. Gilreath. 2010. Relationship of arm span to the effects of prefatigue on performance in the bench press. *The Sport Journal* 22.

Caruso, J.F., S.T. Taylor, B.M. Lutz, N.M. Olson, M.L. Mason, J.A. Borgsmiller, and R.D. Riner. 2012. Anthropometry as a predictor of bench press performance done at different loads. *Journal of Strength and Conditioning Performance* 26 (9): 2460-2467. https://doi.org/10.1519/JSC.0b013e31823c44bb.

Green, C.M., and P. Comfort. 2007. The affect of grip width on bench press performance and risk of injury. *Strength and Conditioning Journal* 29 (5). https://doi.org/10.1519/00126548-200710000-00001.

Grgic, J., B.J. Schoenfeld, T.B. Davies, B. Lazinica, J.W. Krieger, and Z. Pedisic. 2018. Effect of resistance training on gains in muscular strength: A systematic review and meta-analysis. *Sports Medicine* 48:1207-1220. https://doi.org/10.1007/s40279-018-0872-x.

Inklebarger, J., G. Gyer, A. Parkunan, N. Galanis, and J. Michael. 2017. Rotator cuff impingement associated with type III acromial morphology in a young athlete—a case for early imaging. *Journal of Surgical Case Reports* 2017 (1): rjw234. https://doi.org/10.1093/jscr/rjw234.

Keogh, J., P. Hume, P. Mellow, and S. Pearson. 2005. The use of anthropometric variables to predict bench press and squat strength in well-trained strength athletes. International Society of Sports Biomechanics. Proceedings of the 23rd ISBS Conference, Beijing, China, August 22-27.

Krysztofik, M., A. Zajac, P. Zmijewski, and M. Wilik. 2020. Can the cambered bar enhance acute performance in the bench press exercise? *Frontiers in Physiology* 11. https://doi.org/10.3389/fphys.2020.577400.

Lehman, G. 2005. The influence of grip width and forearm pronation/supination on upper-body myoelectric activity during the flat bench press. *Journal of Strength and Conditioning Research* 19 (3): 587-591. https://doi.org/10.1519/R-15024.1.

Lockie, R.G., S.J. Callaghan, A.J. Orjalo, and M.R. Moreno. 2018. Relationships between arm span and the mechanics of the one-repetition maximum traditional and close-grip bench press. *Physical Education and Sport* 16 (2): 271-280. https://doi.org/10.22190/FUPES180525024L.

Lockie, R.G., and M.R. Moreno. 2017. The close-grip bench press. *Strength and Conditioning Journal* 39 (4): 30-35. https://doi.org/10.1519/SSC.0000000000000307.

Newmire, D.E., and D.S. Willoughby. 2018. Partial compared with full range of motion resistance training for muscle hypertrophy: A review and an identification of potential mechanisms. *Journal of Strength and Conditioning Research* 32 (9): 2652-2664.

Rodríguez-Ridao, D., Antequera-Vique, J. A., Martín-Fuentes, I., & Muyor, J. M. (2020). Effect of five bench inclinations on the electromyographic activity of the pectoralis major, anterior deltoid, and triceps brachii during the bench press exercise. *International Journal of Environmental Research and Public Health* 17 (19): 7339.

Swinton, P.A., A.D. Stewart, J.W.L. Keogh, I. Agouris, and R. Lloyd. 2011. Kinematic and kinetic analysis of maximal velocity deadlifts performed with and without the inclusion of chain resistance. *Journal of Strength and Conditioning Research* 25 (11): 3163-3174. https://doi.org/10.1519/JSC.0b013e318212e389.

Chapter 8

Bishop, C., S. Chavda, and A. Turner. 2018. Exercise technique: The push press. *Strength and Conditioning Journal* 40 (3): 104-108. https://doi.org/10.1519/SSC.0000000000000321.

Kraemer, W.J., L.K. Caldwell, E.M. Post, W.H. DuPont, E.R. Martini, N.A. Ratamess, T.K. Szivak, J.P. Shurley, M.K. Beeler, J.S. Volek, C.M. Maresh, J.S. Todd, B.J. Walrod, P.N. Hyde, C. Fairman, and T.M. Best. 2020. Body composition in elite strongman competitors. *Journal of Strength and Conditioning Research* 34 (12): 3326-3330. https://doi.org/10.1519/JSC.0000000000003763.

Pérez, D.V., J.M. Martinez-Sanz, A. Ferriz-Valero, V. Gómez-Vicente, and E. Ausó. 2021. Relationship of limb lengths and body composition to lifting in weightlifting. *International Journal of Environmental Research and Public Health* 18 (2): 756. https://doi.org/10.3390/ijerph18020756.

Saeterbakken, A.H., and M.S. Fimland. 2013. Effects of body position and loading modality on muscle activity and strength in shoulder presses. *Journal of Strength and Conditioning Research* 27 (7): 1824-1831. https://doi.org/10.1519/JSC.0b013e318276b873.

Chapter 9

Dickie, J., J. Faulkner, M. Barnes, and S. Lark. 2017. Electromyographic analysis of muscle activation during pull-up variations. *Journal of Electromyography and Kinesiology* 32: 30-36. https://pubmed.ncbi.nlm.nih.gov/28011412.

Youdas, J.W., C.L. Amundson, K.S. Cicero, J.J. Hahn, D.T. Harezlak, and J.H. Hollman. 2010. Surface electromyographic activation patterns and elbow joint motion during a pull-up, chin-up, or Perfect-Pullup™ rotational exercise. *Journal of Strength and Conditioning Research* 24 (12): 3404-3414.

Chapter 10

Fenwick, C.M.J, S.H.M. Brown, and S.M. McGill. 2009. Comparison of different rowing exercises: Trunk muscle activation and lumbar spine motion, load and stiffness. *Journal of Strength and Conditioning Research* 23 (5): 1408-1417.

Chapter 11

Alahmari, K.A., P. Silvian, S. Reddy, V.N. Kakarparthi, I. Ahmad, and M. Alam. 2017. Hand grip strength determination for healthy males in Saudi Arabia: A study of the relationship with age, body mass index, hand length and forearm circumference using a hand-held dynamometer. *Journal of International Medical Research* 45 (2): 540-548. https://doi.org/10.1177/0300060516688976.

Dhayal, P. 2020. Evaluation of possible anthropometric advantage in sit-up test. *International Journal of Physiology, Nutrition, and Physical Education* 5 (2): 38-42.

Günther, C.M., A. Bürger, M. Rickert, A. Crispin, and C.U. Schulz. 2008. Grip strength in healthy Caucasian adults: Reference values. *Journal of Hand Surgery* 33 (4): 558-565. https://doi.org/10.1016/j.jhsa.2008.01.008.

Howe, L., and P. Read. 2015. Thoracic spine function: Assessment and self-management. *Professional Journal of Strength and Conditioning* 39: 21-30.

McGill, S.M., S. Grenier, N. Kavcic, and J. Cholewicki. 2003. Coordination of muscle activity to assure stability of the lumbar spine. *Journal of Electromyography and Kinesiology* 13 (4): 353-359. https://doi.org/10.1016/S1050-6411(03)00043-9.

Perkilis, K. 2019. Effects of heart rate and blood pressure of weightlifting and breathing technique. *International Journal of Clinical Skills* 13 (1): 254-258.

Rice, V.J., T.L. Williamson, and M. Sharp. 1998. Using anthropometry and strength values to predict grip strength. *Advances in Occupational Ergonomics and Safety: Proceedings of the XIIIth Annual International Occupational Ergonomics and Safety Conference 1998*, 378-381. Japan: IOS Press.

Wilson, J.D., C. Dougherty, M.L. Ireland, and I.S. Davis. 2015. Core stability and its relationship to lower extremity function and injury. *Journal of the American Academy of Orthopaedic Surgeons* 13 (5): 316-325. https://doi.org/10.5435/00124635-200509000-00005.

Chapter 12

Bagchi, A. 2015. A comparative electromyographical investigation of triceps brachii and pectoralis major during four different freehand exercises. *Journal of Physical Education Research* 2 (2): 20-27.

Barakat, C., R. Barroso, M. Alvarez, J. Rauch, N. Miller, A. Bou-Silman, and E.O. De Souza. 2019. The effects of varying glenohumeral joint angle on acute volume load, muscle activation, swelling, and echo-intensity on the biceps brachii in resistance-trained individuals. *Sports* 7 (9): 204. https://doi.org/10.3390/sports7090204.

Barbalho, M., V.S. Coswig, R. Raiol, J. Steele, J.P. Fisher, A. Paoli, A. Bianco, and P. Gentil. 2018. Does the addition of single joint exercises to a resistance training program improve changes in performance and anthropometric measures in untrained men? *European Journal of Translational Myology* 28 (4): 7827. https://doi.org/10.4081/ejtm.2018.7827.

Boland, M.R., T. Spigelman, and T. Uhl. 2008. The function of brachioradialis. *Journal of Hand Surgery* 33 (10): 1853-1859. https://doi.org/10.1016/j.jhsa.2008.07.019.

Da Silva, E.M., Brentano, M.A., Cadore, E.L., De Mameida, A.P., and Martins Kruel, L.F. 2008. Analysis of muscle activation during different leg press exercises at submaximum effort levels. *Journal of Strength and Conditioning Research* 22 (4): 1059-1065. https://doi.org/10.1519/JSC.0b013e3181739445.

de França, H.S., P.A. Nordeste Branco, D.P. Guedes, Jr., P. Gentil, J. Steele, and C.V. La Scala Teixeira. 2015. The effects of adding single-joint exercises to a multi-joint exercise resistance training program on upper body muscle strength and size in trained men. *Applied Physiology, Nutrition, and Metabolism* 40 (8). https://doi.org/10.1139/apnm-2015-0109.

Gentil, P., J. Fisher, and J. Steele. 2017. A review of the acute effects and adaptations of single- and multi-joint exercises during resistance training. *Sports Medicine* 47:843-855.

Kholinne, E., R.F. Zulkarnain, Y.C. Sun, S. Lim, J. Chun, and I. Jeon. 2018. The different role of each head of the triceps brachii muscle in elbow extension. *Acta Orthopaedica et Traumatologica Turcica* 52 (3): 201-205. https://doi.org/10.1016/j.aott.2018.02.005.

Kim, Y.S., D.Y. Kim, and M.S. Ha. 2016. Effect of the push-up exercise at different palmar width on muscle activities. *Journal of Physical Therapy Science* 28 (2): 446-449. https://doi.org/10.1589/jpts.28.446.

Mannarino, P., T. Matta, J. Lima, R. Simão, and B. Freitas de Salles. 2021. Single-joint exercise results in higher hypertrophy of elbow flexors than multijoint exercise. *Journal of Strength and Conditioning Research* 35 (10): 2677-2681. https://doi.org/10.1519/JSC.0000000000003234.

Marcolin, G., N. Petrone, T. Moro, G. Battaglia, A. Bianco, and A Paoli. 2015. Selective activation of shoulder, trunk, and arm muscles: A comparative analysis of different push-up variants. *Journal of Athletic Training* 50 (11): 1126-1132. https://doi.org/10.4085/1062-6050.9.09.

McKenzie, A., Z. Crowley-McHattan, R. Meir, J.W. Whitting, and W. Volschenk. 2021. Glenohumeral extension and the dip: Considerations for the strength and conditioning professional. *Strength and Conditioning Journal* 43 (1): 93-100. https://doi.org/10.1519/SSC.0000000000000579.

Schoenfeld, B., and B. Contreras. 2012. Do single-joint exercises enhance functional fitness? *Strength and Conditioning Journal* 34 (1): 63-65. https://doi.org/10.1519/SSC.0b013e31823e82d7.

van den Tillaar, R. 2019. Comparison of kinematics and muscle activation between pushup and bench press. *International Journal of Sports Medicine* 40 (14): 941-941. https://doi.org/10.1055/a-1021-7893.

Welsch, E.A., Bird, M. and Mahew, J.L.. 2012. Electromyographic activity of the pectoralis major and anterior deltoid muscles during three upper-body lifts. *Journal of Strength and Conditioning Research* 19 (2): 449-452. https://doi.org/10.1519/00124278-2005050000-00034.

About the Authors

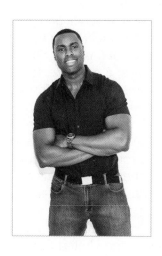

Lee Boyce made the early decision to pursue fitness training as a career while he was still doing his university studies, and he never looked back. He is a strength coach and educator based in Toronto, Canada. He has been helping clients and athletes with strength and conditioning, sport performance, and hypertrophy since 2007. He has developed international recognition as a trainer and as a prolific fitness writer. His expertise has seen him published over 1,200 times by some of the largest publications in the world of fitness and lifestyle media, including *Men's Health*, *Oxygen*, *Train Magazine*, *Inside Fitness*, *Shape*, *Wall Street Journal*, *Huffington Post*, *Men's Journal*, *Esquire*, *Strong Fitness Magazine*, and the National Strength and Conditioning Association's *Personal Training Quarterly*. Lee's first contribution to a full book came in 2013 with his inclusion in *Men's Fitness Exercise Bible: 101 Best Workouts of All Time*, which became an Amazon best seller.

A former national-level university track athlete (sprint and long jump) and kinesiology major, Boyce credits this blend of theoretical and practical experience with his depth of understanding of the human body and biomechanics and his ability to simplify concepts that can be difficult for people to grasp. As a public speaker, Boyce uses his skills to deliver lectures, workshops, and seminars around North America and abroad, sharing innovative troubleshooting guidelines and unique perspectives for trainers looking to improve professionally. As a part-time college professor at Toronto's Humber College, he encourages critical thinking and a departure from the confines of one-size-fits-all, rule-based exercise science advice. It's this type of thinking that developed his passion for speaking and writing about anthropometry and body types as they pertain to resistance training.

Outside of coaching, speaking, writing, and training himself, Lee makes sure he keeps current with his favorite hobby of all time: movies. A book on Lee's favorite films would likely be twice the length of this one.

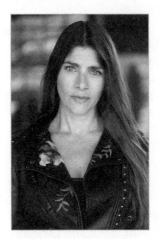

Melody Schoenfeld, MA, CSCS, has well over 27 years of personal training experience and was named National Strength and Conditioning Association's 2019 Personal Trainer of the Year. She is the owner of Flawless Fitness, a small personal training studio located in Pasadena, California. Melody holds a master's degree in health psychology. She has held state and national records in all three lifts in powerlifting (squat, bench press, and deadlift). She competes in strongman, grip sport, and mas wrestling events, and she performs old-time strongman feats of strength such as tearing phone books and bending steel bars.

Her expertise in health and fitness has been featured on numerous television programs throughout the United States, and she has been published and quoted in popular media such as *Shape*, *Oxygen*, *Breaking Muscle*, *Girls Gone Strong*, *My Fitness Pal*, *Men's Fitness*, and *Men's Health*. Melody has several articles published by the *Strength and Conditioning Journal*. She is the author of *Pleasure Not Meating You: A Science-Based Approach to the Vegan Lifestyle (And Some Recipes, Too)* and *Diet Lies and Weight Loss Truths*. Melody speaks nationally and internationally on a wide variety of fitness and nutrition topics. In her spare time, Melody can also be found as the front woman of a number of music groups (mainly heavy metal). When she's not doing all that, she's probably petting a dog somewhere.

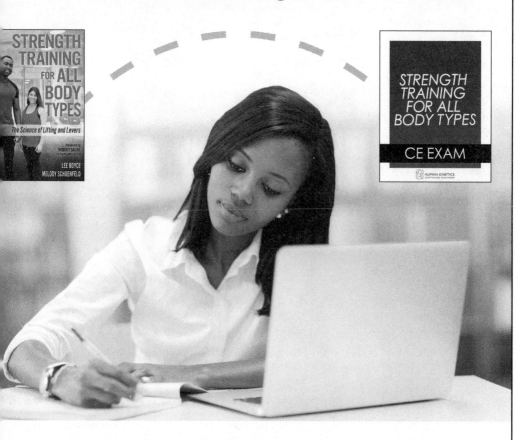
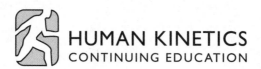

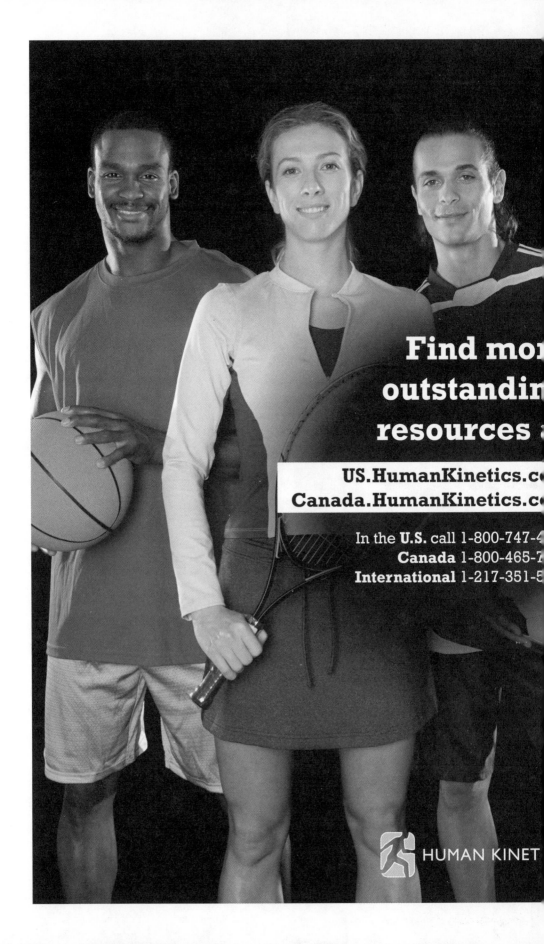